Advanced Praise for Katina I. Makris's
Out of the Woods

"If you or a loved one has Lyme disease you will find yourself resonating with Katina's honest, vivid, and beautifully written prose. Her ability to triumph over this illness and also embrace the journey of personal transformation is a lesson for us all. Out of the Woods *reaches into the core of what true healing fully entails, touching upon life's deepest meanings.*
— Neil Nathan MD
Gordon Medical Associates
Author of Healing is Possible: New Hope for Chronic Fatigue

. . . Lovely, evocative nature writing is interwoven with the accurate portrayal of the insidious onset and, when fully expressed, debilitating impact of the illness on her functioning and how it affected those she loves. Her tale demonstrates that there can be many paths to wellness and that spiritual faith, determination, and a sense of hope can be at least as important to healing as physical "medicaments."
— Kenneth B. Liegner, M.D.

When talking with patients about healing from TBD, I find myself sharing Katina's journey as an example of the way to get their life back. Katina continues to be a beacon of light, encouraging those who are ill and in despair to reach further into themselves to heal all levels of their being—body, mind, and spirit.
— Mara Williams, RN, MSN, ANP-BC, author of Nature's Dirty Needle and founder of Inanna House

Out of the Woods *is as gripping as a novel, smart as the best self-help manuals, and infused with sacred truth as well. This triumphant tale of medical disaster and recovery is much more than exceptionally useful. The author's poetic writing style transforms an already excellent human-interest story into a fountain of profound inspiration. Thousands will read this book seeking information, and end up seeing life in a whole new, healing way.*
— Lonny J. Brown, PhD
Holistic Health Counselor and the author of Enlightenment In Our Time

Lying in bed wondering minute by minute if I am going to make it or not, I couldn't read, watch TV, listen to music, but somehow had a magnetic pull towards this book. Instantly, as I read Katina's story, I felt a mirror of my life which gave me my first sign of hope. Thank you, Katina, for pushing me further into the gift I can now call Lyme to better live each and every day to it's fullest.
— Bethany White Wing
Stylist HBO Productions

For those of us still in the woods, this book is a brilliant ray of hope and inspiration. Have you seen Katina's goddess-like smile and vigor of life? Can you imagine she once was more dead than alive? She is my hero and Out of the Woods *the bible that will lead me back to living.*

—*Sophia Basan*

This book was a game-changer for me. I wish it was available sooner so I could have avoided the damage that antibiotics did to my body. I was inspired by Katina and now am on a more natural path to wellness.

—*Ann Goldman*

Out of the Woods *was the first book I had read after losing my Mom from complications of late stage lyme. It was heartbreaking to read that Katina's story and suffering was similar to my mom's, but I was inspired by Katina's outlook. A true story of hope for anyone battling with this horrendous illness.*

—*Michele and Ken Miller*
Central Mass Lyme Foundation

Out of the Woods *is a must-read for the Lyme affected. Katina Makris eloquently depicts the mind-set, fortitude, and dedication necessary to overcome the chronic form of this illness.*

—*Geordie Thomson, MD*

Like a familiar old friend who understands the journey, this book is a wonderful tool that gives permission to grieve then find your way back to your "new normal." I couldn't stop turning pages."

—*Trish McCleary*
Founder, S.L.A.M. (Sturbridge Lyme Awareness of Massachusetts)

Katina Makris has written a most enlightening book. Her story of regaining her health from chronic Lyme disease is both provocative and deeply meaningful. It touches everyone who has ever faced healing challenges: physical, emotional, or spiritual.

—*Meredith Young-Sowers, DDiv*
Founder and Director, Stillpoint School of Integrative Life Healing, Author,
Agartha: A Journey to the Stars and Spirit Heals: Core Teachings and Practices

A must read for any Chronic Lyme disease sufferer. This book is jam-packed full of honesty, humor, and hope. I read this book during one of my darkest hours. It provided me with that faint glimmer of light at the end of the tunnel, encouraging me to push onward.

—*Christine Moore (misdiagnosed with MS of 18 years)*

Out of the Woods *has saved my life. Without Katina's nurturing words I would still be lost in the throws of Lyme Disease. I thought I could wait to heal my emotions and spirit and just work on the physical ailments. I was so wrong. This book helped me gather the strength to get me on the way back to my life.*

—*Zina Ruben*

I borrowed Out of the Woods *shortly after I was diagnosed with Lyme. It was the first book I read and information I got beside from my doctor. It showed me how serious this disease is and it gave me hope.*

—*Lisa Silver*

Katina offers inspiration and strategies for those dealing with an illness that stumps physicians and scientists alike. While the medical/political debate continues, support for those suffering is few and far between. Katina's message offers encouragement and suggestions that span multiple therapeutic approaches. We need more people speaking up for those who cannot, who remain suffering in isolation from tick-borne illnesses. Katina's intellect and elegance allow her to bring the understanding of this illness to an important tipping point.

—*Susan Nichter*
Professor, Suffolk University

In her riveting personal narrative, Out of the Woods, *Katina powerfully conveys her transformative journey of healing from entrenched misdiagnosed Lyme disease. Katina brings deep knowledge, compassion, and inspiration to those suffering with Lyme disease, a burgeoning worldwide health epidemic. By shining insight on the difficulties in diagnosing and treating this complex and often debilitating illness, Katina offers beacons of hope to those striving to recover and realign body, mind, and spirit.*

—*Nancy Dougherty*
Leadership Gifts Development Officer, The Lyme Disease Research Foundation

Katina is a wonderfully compelling speaker and compassionate author about healing from Lyme disease. Her story is more about winning at life than falling victim to a crippling illness.

—*Robbie Vorhaus*
Author of One Less One More, *CNN, CNBC correspondent, communications strategist, speaker*

Katina Makris is a gifted author and speaker. Once I started reading her book, I couldn't put it down and before I finished it I had booked her for my radio show. She was so well received by my listeners that I invited her back for a second show. She can hold an audience with both her written and spoken words and has something important and interesting to say.

—*Irene Conlan, M.S.N, PH.D*
Host of The Self Improvement Show

Katina Makris tells an important story, especially for those who don't know what living with Lyme is like. And for those who do know about living with Lyme, it is inspirational to know that one can lose it all to Lyme and then reclaim one's life.

—Cynthia Leonard
Rotary Club President, Providence, RI

Without books like this, most lyme-sufferers (after one to two rounds of antibiotics) are condemned to developing what's often (wrongly) labeled fybromyalgia, lupus, and other auto-immune disease, for which doctors have no cure, but which are known to be progressively disabling.Yet, healing is possible! This book gives hope, by way of the author's very own experience and example.

—L. Bauer-Freitag
Author of Healing:The Emerging Holistic Paradigm

This book is giving all of the chronic Lyme community a voice, and giving hope when so many are hopeless.

—Lyme Pixie

Katina does an excellent job with this book relating the story of thousands all over the world suffering from this illness. I realize that people who are not afflicted would never understand the depths of this illness. . . . It is a must read!

—Tessa McCall

This book enlightened and delighted me. It is rare that any author can reach so deeply in the hearts and minds of her readers, and walk them through her journey.Vivid, lucid, beautiful language, a story that so many of use relate to. I laughed, I cried, but lost in her pages, I found hope.

—Alicia Campanella
Florida State National Park Ranger

Out of
the Woods

Healing from Lyme Disease for
Body, Mind, and Spirit

Katina I. Makris, CCH, CIH

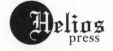

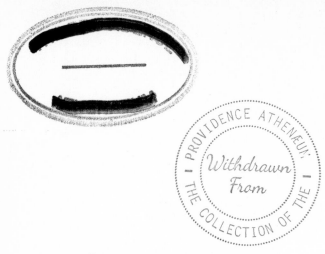

Skyhorse Publishing books may be purchased in bulk at special discounts for sales promotion, corporate gifts, fund-raising, or educational purposes. Special editions can also be created to specifications. For details, contact the Special Sales Department, Helios Press, 307 West 36th Street, 11th Floor, New York, NY 10018 or info@skyhorsepublishing.com.

Helios Press is an imprint of Skyhorse Publishing, Inc.®, a Delaware corporation.

Visit our website at www.skyhorsepublishing.com.

10 9 8 7 6 5 4 3 2 1

Library of Congress Cataloging-in-Publication Data is available on file.

Cover design by Abigail Gehring
Cover image by Thinkstock

ISBN: 978-1-62914-656-0
Ebook ISBN: 978-1-63220-082-2

Printed in the United States of America

Dedication

In the telling of this story, I came to realize how grateful I am for
the deep wellspring of inner resources I bear. I feel the need to honor
my late father, George C. Makris, for instilling me
with a powerful attunement to the gift of resiliency.
I dedicate this book to him.

CONTENTS

Foreword

Lyme disease is the number one spreading vector-borne epidemic worldwide, and mimics common illnesses such as chronic fatigue syndrome/myalgic encephalomyelitis, fibromyalgia, autoimmune diseases like multiple sclerosis, as well as numerous psychiatric disorders. Unreliable blood tests combined with a debate among medical professionals regarding the proper diagnosis and treatment of Lyme disease has resulted in millions of individuals going undiagnosed for long periods of time with disabling symptoms. Patients often tell me the same story. They go to multiple health-care providers looking for answers for their chronic fatigue, migratory joint and muscle pain, nerve pain, headaches, insomnia, and memory/concentration problems. They ultimately discover after years of suffering with debilitating symptoms, oftentimes resulting in losing their faculties and jobs, and disrupting their relationships with family and friends, that Lyme and associated tick-borne diseases were responsible for their illness.

Out of the Woods gives hope and inspiration to those affected by this epidemic. Patients often tell me of their confusion, despair, and broken spirit after being told that there is nothing wrong with them, and that it is all "in their head." Katina's story of using her life-altering struggles with Lyme disease as a healing journey helps us to see how difficult circumstances can be transformed, and how a deep commitment to healing can end in triumph. With eloquence, bravery, and intimate honesty, this is a heartwarming story with glimpses into how working with the mind, body, and spirit can help us to transform our experience into one of personal growth and, ultimately, success.

Dr. Richard Horowitz, February 5, 2014
Hyde Park, NY

Author of *Why Can't I Get Better?*
Solving the Mystery of Lyme and Chronic Disease

Founding Member of ILADS

Preface

I first stumbled across Lyme disease in the mid-1990s, while practicing medicine in Springfield, Missouri. A few patients came into my office with odd, almost inexplicable symptoms: overwhelming fatigue, intense cognitive impairment ("brain fog"; loss of memory, concentration, and focus), numbness and tingling in places that did not make sense from a strictly neurological description, headaches, joint and muscle pain, muscle spasms and twitches, incapacitating anxiety and depression, stomach pains with nausea and vomiting, unusual visual impairments, heart palpitations, and specific symptoms suggesting compromise of specific nerves. These unfortunate individuals had seen lots of specialists, and were told repeatedly that these symptoms matched no known medical condition—so they were offered medications for anxiety and depression and sent off to suffer.

Working in the field of integrative, holistic medicine, I became aware that rumors of a newly discovered condition called Lyme disease had begun to circulate. At that time, medical science and specialists were of little help in making that diagnosis. The only tests that even hinted at the presence of Lyme disease were the Western blot test and later the CD 57, both of which are, at best, indirect suggestions that Lyme disease is even possible. So we were left with the options of allowing these patients to deteriorate, untreated, or trying to use massive doses of antibiotics in the hope that we would see improvement over time. For a holistic physician, it was a difficult decision to contemplate the use of long-term antibiotics without guarantee of success, but what other choices did we have?

To make this a bit dicier, virtually all of the infectious disease specialists who practiced in my area categorically denied the existence of Lyme disease. Despite the fact that the State Department of Health published regular material documenting hundreds of cases of Lyme disease, the specialists maintained that they had never seen a case.

So, with minimal support from the medical profession or laboratories, we were faced with a growing tide of patients who came to us for help. For most of them, the antibiotics worked, often only after months, even years, of treatment, and most of my patients improved or recovered completely. It was obvious to me that this condition was real and treatable. More and more patients found their way to my office and I had to learn more about it.

It turned out that Lyme disease was perhaps the most complicated infection we had ever seen. You may not be aware of this, but most bacteria have the ability to change their structure when they are threatened by the host's defense system or antibiotics—and it turns out that the Lyme bacteria, which is a spirochete (similar to syphilis), can change back and forth from its customary spiral bacterial structure to a cell-wall-deficient structure to a microscopic cyst structure, to literally hide from the immune system or antibiotics. This means that treatment often requires chasing these changes because different antibiotics are necessary for each different structure.

If that weren't bad enough, it has become clear that this bacteria is not the only infectious agent injected into the body when bitten by a tick—other bacteria, notably *Bartonella* and *Mycoplasma*, can be acquired at the same time, as can the parasite *Babesia*, which is in the malaria family.

If that weren't bad enough, the weakening of the immune system deliberately caused by these infectious microbes allows previously dormant infections like viruses and chlamydia to reactivate, so that we now have a virtual cesspool of insidious microbes competing with each other for a piece of the host's body, creating a maelstrom of infectious activity and setting off a profound release of inflammatory cytokines that the host desperately produces to try to deal with this, further contributing to the profoundly debilitating symptoms already set in motion.

As more and more patients found the few physicians willing to try to come to grips with this complexity, we learned a lot more about things we needed to be aware of to improve our treatment. It became clear that it was not enough to give the correct antibiotics, but that we also had to provide support for the body's ability to detoxify the waste products of the battle it was waging with these bugs because it turned out that those waste products produced similar symptoms to the diseases themselves! It also turned out that these toxins, as well as the infections themselves, inflamed the brain and pituitary gland, compromising the ability of the adrenals, thyroid, and sex hormones to function properly, adding even more symptoms and complexity to our treatment plan.

So, fast-forward to 2014, now. The CDC has just announced that it had seriously underestimated the number of patients now suffering from chronic Lyme disease, admitting to at least three hundred thousand. While those of us who work in this field suspect this to be a very low estimate, at least one major health authority has at last announced that this is real, and it is officially an epidemic. We still do not have a decent test for the co-infections of *Bartonella*, *Babesia*, or their cousins. For example, there are twenty-seven known strains of *Bartonella*, and we have tests for only two of them. There are one hundred six known strains of *Babesia*, and we have tests for only two of them. Even for Lyme disease itself, we have now clearly identified several species of bacteria that are more common than we have thought, and we had no commercial tests for those, either.

Lyme disease might be the most controversial disease of our generation (competing with autism, chronic fatigue syndrome, and fibromyalgia for that honor). Experts disagree as to what it is, what causes it, and how to treat it, leaving patients holding the proverbial bag. Insurance companies have used this controversy to deny treatment coverage, making the expensive antibiotic and herbal treatment programs a very expensive out-of-pocket process. As patients with this bewildering array of symptoms present themselves for diagnosis, the lack of agreement, or awareness, on the part of the medical profession has led to years of going from specialist to specialist with no diagnosis and no treatment. By the time we finally see these patients, they have exhausted their finances and are usually on disability, as they have not been able to work for quite some time. If all of this sounds pretty awful, there is no way around that fact—it is.

There are quite a few good books that can help these unfortunate patients learn about Lyme disease and how to treat it properly, covering many of the areas I have alluded to above.

However, the emotional and spiritual components of the illness have not received the same attention. What makes this book so special is that Katina has shared the intimate aspects of her journey with you. Her beautiful, graphic descriptions of her emotional roller-coaster ride will help thousands of others to know that they are not alone in their suffering. The profound, inexplicable sudden shifts from intense, incapacitating anxiety to the depths of despair are extremely common and affect most of our patients. The intensity of these feelings, and the sense of feeling completely out of control, at times even crazy, are almost universal.

I have encouraged all of my patients to read this book as a way of both understanding what is happening to them and to know that indeed, others have had similar experiences and found a way to get through this to reach health again.

One under-appreciated part of this journey is that this is an overwhelming illness—it causes profound fatigue and exhaustion and severe cognitive impairment and anxiety and depression and pain—so that it literally takes over the lives of those who have it, and the lives of their families who are trying to be helpful, but do not know how to do that. For those who suffer from Lyme disease and its co-infections, it is difficult to escape from the reality that this has taken over their lives, and they begin to live the life of illness. After even a few years, their lives, and those of their families, become consumed by this illness.

Here again, Katina's brave description of the spiritual component of her journey can serve as a road map toward health. It is a critical part of treatment that patients understand that they can get well, but it usually will require both emotional and spiritual bravery to face their inner demons and doubts and fears, what St. John described as the "dark night of the soul."

For those with the courage to make this journey, we have found that many rediscover the essence of themselves and find meaning in this process. I believe it is important to find the personal meaning of this illness for each person who has it, to reframe the disease not as a dark, meaningless void, but as an opportunity for growth and awareness. Those who have done so are never the same. Their compassion and empathy for others has grown exponentially.

So, brave person, I commend you for picking up this book. If you or a loved one has Lyme disease, you will find yourself resonating with Katina's honest, vivid, and beautifully written prose. Her ability to triumph over this illness and also embrace the journey of personal transformation is a lesson for us all. *Out of the Woods* reaches into the core of what true healing fully entails, touching upon life's deepest meanings. It is my hope it will help you to understand what is happening to you and to know that you are not alone.

My deepest wishes for a successful journey,

Neil Nathan, MD
Gordon Medical Associates
Author of *Healing Is Possible: New Hope for Chronic Fatigue, Fibromyalgia, Persistent Pain, and Other Chronic Illnesses*

Acknowledgments

My own spiritual awakening and inner discoveries thumped within, urging me to share the story of *Out of the Woods*. But how to begin, with my writer's voice long silenced by the muddy vortex of illness?

In the summer of 2007 I joined a writers' group. My first sessions, sitting amid a dozen prosaic scribes left me in a stew of confusion. Strangled words and images clotted about in my mind. Completely daunted I also felt inspired to try and capture my own mirages.

The group leader provided various prompts for each time-blocked writing unit. A feather placed in my outstretched palm or a cluster of vintage props sprawled on the barn floor before us eked remote memories or snippets of cloudy vignettes from me. Still very fragile, my hand shook a mere twenty minutes into a session. But, doggedly I held on.

On a sultry July day, a Mary Oliver quote was read aloud: "*As you strode deeper and deeper into the world, determined to do the only thing you can do, determined to save the only life you can save . . .*" Something clicked open within me—a flashback! I was ascending a hemlocked mountain trail, my faithful dog at my side, the colors, scents, foliage cascading through me. Effortlessly, I recreated this pinnacle day on paper. Reading "Mastering the Mountain" aloud to the group, my voice felt sure.

"Keep going!" the others urged, "You've got something there."

Over the ensuing weeks a dozen more scenes, the backbone of this book, were birthed. The cherished antique barn we gathered in added enough magic to stir my muse from hiding. Soon enough, I knew I had it—this story, a talisman of hope in hand, and a toolbox of healing resources to share. For three years I kept at it.

Gratitude has a strong presence in my life. Every day I give thanks for the bounty of gifts in my world. I could not have made this journey or published *Out of the Woods* without the assistance of so many invaluable people. I want to acknowledge the efforts of my helpmates.

Dawson Church, my initial publisher at Elite Books, you believed in this book and my message from the get-go. It is still a marvel to me how you plucked *Out of the Woods* from a swell of manuscripts on your desk one February day. Thank you for giving this book its wings. To my Elite Books editor, Courtney Arnold, your intelligence and hand-holding make you a publishing midwife extraordinaire! Our bi-coastal bond holds fast.

To my ever alert agent Dede Cummings, thank you for taking this lovely tale and bringing it to the big leagues. You are so close to my spirit.

Abigail Gehring, my editor at Skyhorse Publishing, you are a joy and so supportive of this subject and understand the destruction Lyme creates. Thank you for understanding my gifts and giving me an opportunity to inspire the world. Your team has been truly patient and enduring!

Kate Gleason, writing group svengali and my first read through editor deserves special accolades. You stirred the seed of conception and your poetic sensitivity made me believe in this story. Thank you.

My fellow group writers the summer of 2007, circling together in Mimi Bull's barn, held me in a web of creative promise. I appreciate your encouragement and devotion to our craft. Synergy cannot be dismissed.

Suzanne Kingsbury, you are like a sister to me! How miraculous that you read this book and wrote me to become your healer and friend. And now, you are so dear to my heart and hold me in such enriching creativity as Gateless Writing Salon group leader and editor. Bless you and Peter, forever, in those scary summer nights that I flew to you and for encouraging me to take this book to the next level.

Technical advice came from the willing support of Dr. Sarah Featherstone, Dr. Ahmed Kilani at Clonegen Labs, and Dr. Nick Harris at Igenex Labs. My great appreciation for your time and knowledge.

Dee McGrath-Fischer once said to me, "don't forget the little people," her twinkling smile lighting the room, as yet she printed out another draft of the book for me. Truly Dee, no one is "little" to me. Each of you is great, no matter how minor or major your role has been. Favored thanks to you all—an extra dose to Paulette McAlexander.

My tarot queens, Nell Conkright, Joanie Packzowski, Tracy Hedberg, and Amelia Shea provided me with wise council. Thank you for fanning the embers of my dreams.

As *Out of the Woods* birthed a new pathway for me, I traveled the country bringing in education, inspiration, and hope for recovery. My assistants have been youthful, hardworking allies, keeping me organized and fueled on my mission. Without your fabulous abilities to learn on the curve, be upbeat and social media savvy, I would not be where I am today! My appreciation of each of you is eternal. Thank you Carrie Dumas, Stephanie Kamp, Charlotte Miller, and Catherine Bailey. We have had enormous fun, too! Extra blessings to Arianna Meehan for the long editorial hours we pulled at midnights and your kindred spirit. And, Xtophr Talon, major thanks for the protection.

I thank the Lyme disease community at large. This self-made network of scientists, healthcare providers, activists, cutting-edge laboratories, stricken individuals, authors, and support groups intimately know the convoluted maelstrom this spirochete bacteria induces. The agony, the madness, the sheer confusion of Lyme disease must be amended. I applaud the endless work and compassion so many of you devote. You are relentlessly working to shift the tides of an overlooked public health care crisis. At grassroots levels and on tiny budgets you brave people never loose sight of what matters the most—preventing more damage. You are embedded in my heart, as we forge through treacherous waters to help others.

My dear friends at Tick Borne Disease Alliance—David Roth, John Donnally, Jodi Nass, Charles Balducci, Staci Grodin—thank your for going to bat with me on so many collaborative venues. Aligned together, we can make a difference.

I must say that the three years out on the road speaking to folks in all sorts of gatherings, from rallies, to galas, to music festivals, book stores, and Lyme support groups, I have tasted and smelled the breadth and depth of the Lyme disease epidemic and it is *not* good! However, the kindness you have all showed me is touching, as I sleep in your homes, you ferry me to speaking engagements, and create space for me to bring in healing. I feel a palpable kinship in our mutual understandings of the suffering and the valiant efforts to bring about change. Thank you truly for all the care you give me as I come to your communities and for your terrific organizational skills making events happen. I have new friends in every part of the world!

The absolutely sterling health care providers I have met and worked with in these years are breathtaking. The list is too long to state, but let me say that the bravery, open-mindedness, and true compassion of these individuals (many ILADS members) is saving lives every single minute. Many of you have battled politically, fought to retain your license to practice, and gone out on a limb to minister to those maimed in this epidemic. I bow to you all, for you are heroes in a very dark time in our lives. Heartfelt thanks to Dr Ricard Horowitz, Dr Kenneth Liegner, Dr. Neil Nathan, Mara Williams, and Dr Tom Francescott for working individually with me as we educate.

To my fabulous team at Transformation Talk Radio—you all *rock*! Dr Pat Bacilli, Linda Firing, Jesica Henderson, Chris DiPaulo, Brian Sullivan—each week we bring cutting edge information and guests to millions world wide on "Lyme Light Radio with Katina." What an honor to host this show and shine a light on such a critical topic.

And to Gregg Kirk, the founder of the Ticked OFF Music Fest series, your friendship, your belief in my message, and our collaborative energy is life altering for thousands. You have helped give this book a new trajectory and my voice a powerful conduit.

The physicians and healers in my complicated Lyme journey tended to my body, my psyche, and my heart. Each one of you has been indispensable and at times frank lifelines. True gratitude to Geordie Thomson, MD, Lisa Ramey, MD, Jeffrey Sullander, CCn—your seasoned knowledge changed the course of my life.

Acupuncturists Marilyn Morgan,LicAc, Deborah Meuse,Lic Ac, Yilin Ma,LicAc—many thanks for ushering me over some jagged mountain passes. Vic Pantesco, EDD, and Dr. Catherine Cauthorne,Ph.D, thank you for soothing my jangled mind and the scars of trauma.

My body workers are still my bedrock. Vinnie Procitta, DC, Aaron Bard, DC, John Lunan, Lynn Ann Palmer, Bruce Birenbaum, Lonny Brown, Ildi Ingraham, Alex Walker—I appreciate your talents and caring.

Homeopathy is woven into my soul. This healing art is like no other—acutely sensitive, yet powerful. Dear Savitri Clarke,CCH, Lic Ac, I bow to you and my masterful homeopathic teachers over the decades.

To my beloved spiritual mentor, Meredith Young-Sowers,Dr. Div— I offer you everlasting gratitude. Your guidance and love helped me reclaim my life and enhanced my abilities to help others heal. And, to the Stillpoint family, I offer utmost respect from my deep heart.

My friends are true angels. Many times I felt I could not possibly survive if it were not for your help. I thank you for the grocery shopping, the errands, the packing and unpacking, the chauffeuring, the childcare, the tear-filled talks, and your profound kindness. Allen, I leaned on you so strongly. Thank you for the support and for all you do for the children.

Family means so much to a woman of Mediterranean roots like me. My indomitable Aunt Vangie, thank you for helping through some very tenuous stretches. Barbara, my dear sister, you believed in me no matter how dire things looked on the outside. Thank you for holding the faith. To the Barrows and Sawyer clans thank you for "taking me in." Darling Rachel, you are a gem, bringing sunshine into my life. Shine on! To my brilliant Jake, I give my heart. It is because of you and our amazing closeness that I refused to give in to the illness. You hold the family legacy. Thank you, honey.

And finally, I thank my angels and guides in the natural world and spirit realm. I feel your presence and protection often at the most unsuspect hour, under the hush of the evening sky, or perhaps dancing on the sunlight sparkles of the pond.

Namaste.

Katina I. Makris, CCH, CIH

Introduction

Thousands of people are afflicted with chronic Lyme disease. Thousands more are wrongly diagnosed with illnesses such as fibromyalgia, lupus, chronic fatigue syndrome, rheumatoid arthritis, and more, when in actuality the Lyme microbes are at the root of their problems. Mysterious symptoms, alarming fatigue, and an unexplained ability to get well accompany these omnipresent struggles. Lyme disease can be a misleading and devastating illness when neglected or misdiagnosed, leading to sometimes life-altering effects. Once considered to be a short-term infectious illness, the past two decades of patient results and clinical findings have illuminated that chronic Lyme disease is a multifaceted, complex, systemic illness of a treacherous nature. Recovery is often only partial, if not addressed thoroughly.

This country is currently in the throes of a swiftly moving explosion of Lyme disease. Thousands of cases are contracted weekly and the population of the tick that is the primary carrier is multiplying in far greater proportions than has been historically normal. One esteemed doctor I encountered compares Lyme's rapid growth to that of the polio epidemics of the last century. Immediate attention, funding, research, and doctoring needs to be put into stepped- up action mode regarding diagnosis and treatment of Lyme disease.

A big problem is that large sectors of the medical community are uninformed about the extent of chronic Lyme, its various forms, and even proper laboratory diagnostic and treatment routes. Much controversy abounds surrounding the chronic form of Lyme disease, as the Centers for Disease Control has yet to establish criteria for long-term infections, leaving many physicians in the dark about making a proper diagnosis. The conventional ELISA and Western blot Lyme test panels will not necessarily identify a case of chronic Lyme disease, merely an early onset case. This is the first hurdle that needs to be surmounted within our medical arena, utilizing more refined testing techniques to achieve an adequate diagnosis.

In the pages ahead you will read the true story of my own battle with Lyme disease. On a sublime summer's day a mysterious "flu" entered my life, eroding all that I had worked so hard to build and cherish. I was happily ensconced in the rural beauty of New Hampshire, with a successful homeopathic practice and popular newspaper health column. My young family, husband, and I would suffer mighty blows from several doctors' misdiagnoses and their lack of information. During these enormously trying times I discovered much about myself, humankind, chronic illness, and the power of hope. As a veteran health-care practitioner, I was seasoned in the art of helping others to heal. The circumstances I faced were entirely overwhelming, however. The hidden Lyme experience asked me to turn within and find ways to heal myself. Like Persephone, my journey into the underworld of my life and back to the light of living has been one of profound discoveries and a spiritual awakening I could not have conjured on my own.

Please note that the names of nearly all people and places have been changed in this story in an effort to maintain anonymity. The name of cofounder and director of the Stillpoint School of Integrative Life Healing, Dr. Meredith Young-Sowers, has not been altered, however, as I consider her remarkable work and her unique school too important to be camouflaged. Please note that my given name is Katina Irene Makris. My nickname, Kim, is derived from my initials.

I extend to you this story of mine from a place of true inner healing. I feel this evolution through Lyme disease has served a purpose in my life. One obvious one is that I share the intrinsic pieces that helped me recover. Another is to illuminate the important facets of emotional and spiritual recovery, which can apply to all forms of serious illness. Without being emotionally, spiritually, and physically whole, we cannot be well.

It's my wish to bear a flame of illumination in the tragically darkened hours of your night. There is wisdom banked in the quiet reaches of your soul. We are all entwined together as beings in this cosmos of living. Whether it be this story of mine, the smile of a trusted friend, or a message drifting to you on the thermals of a summer sky, there is promise for your healing. But you do need to reach out, search, and ask for guidance as I did in my bleakest despair. The answers will arise. Listen for them, follow your instincts, embrace your own knowing. Your true inner healing will come.

Blessings to you,
Katina I. Makris, CCH, CIH
New Hampshire
Spring 2015

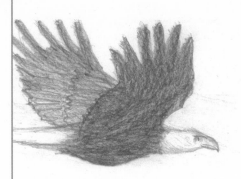

PART ONE

Out of the Woods— A Memoir

"Come to the edge," he said.
"We are afraid," they replied.
"Come to the edge," he said.
They did.
He pushed them and they flew.

—Guillaume Apollinaire

Prologue

The evening sky speaks in quiet shades of rose and gold, as the final hush of twilight fades on the horizon. A butternut glow, dipping beyond the sleeping hills, leaves behind the final silent traces of daylight's streaming sun. I see the first twinkle of the evening star peeking above the stately old pines, reminding me that yet another world is about to dawn—that of the night, the time of mystery and charms, passions and dreams. I sit by the campfire embers, relishing the good fortune in my world.

It has been a glorious summer day on the lake—a day of beauty, laughter, and play to be banked in my memories as a time of bliss. I am at peace, happy to share with my family, to love with an open heart, and to bask in the glory of union. I see vibrant greens and clear blues in bold swatches, as the laughter of children and calls of the white-throated sparrow pepper the air. High-pitched, shrill giggles and lanky limbs flail wildly off the fraying rope swing. Voluminous splashes into icy cold water and scrambles up the rocky perch to arch once again over the lake in another fit of rambunctious fun. Chattering teeth, sopping hair, and exhilaration wrap the buoyant face of each child awaiting a turn on Old Yeller, the mighty rope swing.

The sturdy, aged limb of a granddaddy oak tree has lent itself to uncountable summers of thrills, at the back corner of Lake Pomequit. Tucked amongst spruce and maples and huge stands of mountain laurel, Old Yeller proudly raises his wizened limbs high and broad over the tranquil waters. A few decades back a band of kids anointed Old Yeller with the legendary title of King of the Rope Swings. As long as his stalwart limbs hold strong, Old Yeller will baptize many a child into the ritual fun of hot summer days, the freedom of open skies, swarming dragonflies, and fresh air rippling across the lake.

Old Yeller bears a long tradition of daring. Generations of children have tested themselves by holding fast to Old Yeller's heavy rope, digging their toes into the bumpy backbone of the gray granite boulder, and pushing forth in a burst of energy. They fling themselves far enough out above the water, over the deepest part, to then bravely let go, rocketing into the unknown depths. It's dark. It's quiet. It's sublimely secretive under there. Surging upward, with all their might, and reaching for air in a sudden, startling breath, it's a heady grin on the face that we onlookers see as a swimmer busts forth, brimming with the power of it all. And then, the call to *do it again!*

One must come by canoe or boat or swim across to Old Yeller; he is not availed by land. This section of lake and woods is protected as conservation property. It's pristine and magical. I can't help but feel the shadows of Native inhabitants sheltered in these dense woodlands, where they fished and hunted amongst the thronging wildlife. Their ghosts are palpable to me, as if they are not far off, perhaps tending to a campfire or baby. I feel their footfalls in these humble hills, moccasined feet walking softly through the hemlocked glades.

Once upon a time, as an Indian princess in my tomboy childhood, I fantasized of a life in the deep woods, along the wending rivers. I spent many hours reading *The Leatherstocking Tales*, cherishing the details of Mohican life and the fearless scout Hawkeye. It only makes sense that time would pass and I would gravitate to a man who felt the course of a cresting river as a pulse in his veins.

Sometimes I see my husband at an odd angle, and he looks to me like a Canadian trapper of yore, paddling the networking lakes and rivers of the Hudson Bay, fur pelts stacked along the gunnels of his boat. The tilt of his head, the broad sweep of his strong back, the power with which he drives the canoe through the current speaks to me of something other than now. I see Joel in heavy woolen clothing and fur-muffed hats, with a firm determination to soldier through any wicked spate of weather. Joel's dark hair and certain brow make sense to me here on the backwaters. It's as if a French Canadian bloodline runs through him, though in reality he is of eastern European and old Spanish Sephardic ancestry.

Back in modern society Joel manifests as the charmer, the intelligent bon vivant, with a laugh and a joke, and a quick dance step. He is a successful businessman, a devoted father. Out here, however, mixed in with babbling streams and lapping waves, Joel seems more relaxed. The veneer drops, his confidence soars. He's indomitable, a force to be reckoned with. I trust him with my life.

Joel and I work together with skill—navigating, paddling, portaging our family, our ideals, and our love of the outdoors in our sleek green canoe. Sleeping under the starlight, we listen to the owls hoot in their mating parlance. This lake is a place of great beauty, known for its cool, deep, pure water. We play on the elephant-sized collective of boulders, climbing up their heaving curves, to survey the perimeter of the lake. A mere spattering of isolated homes dot a scant pocket of shoreline. Otherwise, it's untouched by man, a step back in time.

As I take in the glory of the twilight sky by our campfire, I watch Sarah and Eli play along the shoreline, dashing along the water's edge collecting pinecones and pebbles.

"Fire's ready, kids," I call. "Let's cook the marshmallows."

I watch their light-filled faces as they race toward us, dampened hair and wide smiles carving crescents of love in my heart. I look to Joel and recognize a swell of pride and contentedness in the laughing corners of his hazel eyes.

"They're so beautiful," I say softly to him.

"Yes," he says, as he reaches out to hold my hand, "and so free."

Summer Solstice

I wake rosy-cheeked Eli from his nap, the afternoon sunshine streaming in the south windows of his bedroom. My three-year-old son's sleep-dampened curls press delicately against my neck as we descend the stairs, Eli, astride my hip, still groggy with dreams.

It is a beautiful summer solstice, June 21, 2000. New England summertime at its best, I think. The last few days have been postcard perfect: clear air, crystalline skies, and wildflowers bursting in color. I love late June especially, for its lush green forests and long leisurely hours of daylight. We all savor these precious months, especially in counterpoint to the fierce New Hampshire winters.

"Joel, I've got to go. Can you take Eli?" I call as I walk outside onto the deck where he sits with Sarah.

"Sure, here." Joel extends his arms upward, Eli tipping downward onto his daddy's lap.

"I've got to get over to the Hawthornes'. It's the last hour of Wyeth's vigil."

"No problem," Joel says.

"Can you get dinner started? There's fish in the fridge," I suggest.

"Sure, easy enough."

"Shoo! Bombay, shoo!" I blurt out, flicking my arm in the direction of one of our backyard hens, her head craned upward toward Sarah's cracker-filled hand. How bold these girls can get, creeping up on the deck searching for crumbs.

"Bad Bombay," Eli announces, grinning slyly, as he, too, tosses a tiny hand in her direction, mimicking me. Bombay retreats to the lawn and the rest of the flock, while Echo, our eager border collie, moves into herding stance.

"Gotta go," I say, as I kiss a good-bye to each family member.

Sarah swivels the outdoor rocking chair in circles.

"I'll be home by six," I call over my shoulder, as I skim out the sun-room door. "Love you."

I navigate the back roads with ease. These parts are so familiar to me now. I pass the entrance to one of my favorite hikes, an old, over-grown cart path. The sun-dappled trail beckons and I think instantly of dear Wyeth, who was so at home in the woods. What a shame that he is gone.

Wyeth Hawthorne was a weathered sprite of a man, an intuitive, and skilled in the ways of the land. A throwback to eras past, he was an Earthwright by trade, dowsing for wells, laying out sacred labyrinths, and reading the terrain for the best placements of a house site. Sadly, we lost Wyeth unexpectedly in a swift landslide to leukemia. His sudden decline caught us all by surprise.

On my last walk in the woods with Wyeth, we visited a favored spot, an outcropping of stately granite boulders clumped at the end of an untouched pond. We sat in silence for some time, meditating on the magic of our natural kingdom and its vast powers. We watched wood ducks squawk and climb in flight, then the arrival of a flock of Canadian geese, tawny downed goslings trailing in tow, paddling in single file. Their curious black eyes peered up at us, questioning these large gangly creatures resting on the rocks.

Wyeth told me he had seen glimpses of the "other side" as of late. He knew his time to pass was coming. He was weak and frail, nearing the end of his earth days. It was a poignant visit, saying my good-bye to this unusual man who walked amid the trees and hills as if he knew their heartbeats like his own. Wyeth had sensed my own earth-centered proclivities over the years, teaching me how to read the weather and a cluster of trees gathered in a ring, and to play the didgeridoo.

Today, at the Hawthornes', I sit with Wyeth's deceased body for one hour as his family has designed. His numerous friends and loved ones each take a turn being with him, as his spirit ascends in these days after death. The instructions are to sit in prayer or meditation, or to read to him from one of a stack of books—Thoreau, Emerson, Mary Oliver—easing his crossing, paying our respects. It's a thoughtful hour for me, both sad and contemplative. Flowers, cards, ribbons, drawings, and candles are everywhere, surrounding the altar near his casket. Much love and familial outpouring flows in the home.

In these minutes with Wyeth much runs through my mind. I reflect on the rich life he lived and the palpable truth that I will miss him. Death has a way of making me grateful for what I have, a reminder to cherish my family, our sturdy oaken home in the countryside, and my health. It reminds me to honor my ancestors, to recognize how hard we have each worked to get where we are today. I feel a great reverence within.

Sitting with Wyeth in these moments, I feel the gossamer veil between the worlds part and open, gathering in this dear soul, but also whispering a warning to me, of a tumultuous storm on my horizon. In my mind's eye I see brooding, dark towers of clouds and hurricane-force winds ahead. A frightening hum covers my skull. In earnest, I will this picture out of my mind and try to stay present with Wyeth.

The ebbing afternoon sunshine, illuminating the west windows, is soft and enveloping and feels nicer to me than the storm in my head. But when I rise to depart, saying good-bye to Wyeth's family members, an overwhelming rush of dizziness, heaviness, and nausea floods me. Is it my emotional state, the air being too still, or perhaps me being hungry? I realize I need some air and hastily manage to express my sentiments to Wyeth's wife before going.

"Lynn, I'm so sorry Wyeth's gone. He was such a special man. So poetic in his knowings and patient with us all. I'll miss him. I know how hard it must be for each of you."

"Thank you, Kim, for the kindness. Your homeopathic remedies helped us."

I sense an inner strength in her that I would be proud to claim as my own during such a time. But my head is swimming, my throat burning raw in pain. I express my condolences to the others and quickly plunge for the outside fresh air, my car awaiting me in the descending twilight.

On the drive home I feel just awful. Chills creep up my spine and neck, a clammy, feverish moisture clings to my brow, and muscle pains wrap around my shoulders and down the sides of my legs. I'm thinking that a summertime flu is sometimes worse than a wintertime one, as it seems so wrongly placed on a breezy, sunny day.

As I round the bend in the road, toward the climb over Arrow Mountain homeward, the dizziness floods me again, this time like a tidal wave. I have to pull over to steady myself and let my vision clear. Swollen glands, intensely sore throat, emerging headache. I figure a client in my office must have brought this flu bug in the door to me. By the time I get home, I feel like hell.

Standing at the kitchen sink, doing after-dinner dishes and watching the kids playing in the yard outside the double-hung windows, I call out to Joel, asking him to go upstairs to my homeopathic home pharmacy and get a bottle of gelsemium, a remedy that can often halt flu dead in its tracks. I start popping the pellets and dowse myself with a sturdy dose of zinc and echinachea, hoping to kick this thing out before it grabs hold too fiercely.

"Go up to bed early, Kim," Joel says. "I'll get the kids tucked in."

By 7:30 I'm under the covers, aching and perspiring, determined to sweat this thing out while I sleep.

As dawn breaks, I'm surprised to find I feel just as horrid. Homeopathic remedies and a quick jump on vitamins usually curtail any common illness in me. With my unusually strong immune system, I rarely pick up typical colds and flus. I have never had bronchitis, strep, or pneumonia in my life. Now, I have to call clients and cancel my day at the office.

Three days later I'm no better, even weaker, in fact. Strangely, the flu has not progressed into the typical respiratory symptoms. I muster up enough self-will to get to the office and see people. After the first client, though, my head is whirling. I can barely concentrate. Objects appear to be moving around the room. My head feels as if a boulder is bearing down on it. I don't believe I've ever felt this sick in my life. I stumble downstairs into the office of my former business partner, John Miller, MD.

"John, something is terribly wrong with me," I grumble. "I'm totally woozy and so much aches, everywhere."

John gives me a quick exam, has some blood work ordered, and insists I cancel clients and go back to bed for two days. He loads me up with some good immune-support herbs.

"But we have to take Sarah up to sleepaway camp tomorrow in Vermont," I moan. "It's her first time away from home, and it's this special camp I went to as a kid, too. It's a tradition in my family. I have to go help her get settled in."

"No," he tells me. "Your blood pressure is off, you've got swollen glands, and your complexion is gray. I don't want you going anywhere." John levels me with a look. "Stay home," he says.

In the morning I leave for camp, against John's wishes. Most of the day is a hallucinatory blur. I feel disconnected from my body, as if riding on the ceiling of the car. Joel makes me a blanket nest to rest on in the backseat of the van. Sarah rides up front, next to Eli in his car seat.

I adored my summers at the Maidenwood Camps. I want to help Sarah get off to a good start. I hope she will find as much love, camaraderie, and adventure there as I did. At ten years old, Sarah is bravely venturing off without a buddy in tow, trusting my words of encouragement after a brief preview visit last summer. I want to share this entryway in life with her. But, geez, do I feel crappy!

As we pull into the Dolphin Dell, where all the ten-year-olds live for their stay at Maidenwood, I smell the same familiar blend of pine pitch and driveway tar from thirty years ago. My heart sings in happiness for the fun awaiting Sarah. Memories of s'mores, sailing on soft lake breezes, and singing at evening circle return to my mind. We settle Sarah into her platform tent, a family of three campers and counselor, smiling brightly.

The next morning, I wake up at home, feeling horrid and unable to remember anything else from our camp drop-off with Sarah. I must have slept the whole trip back.

"Something is way wrong with me," I tell Joel. "I should've listened to John."

"You'll see him tomorrow," Joel says. "He should have the blood work results by then."

I sleep the rest of the day in fitful sweats.

"You're dehydrated and have a mild bacterial infection," John says when I see him. "Maybe a sinus infection or a respiratory infection," he concludes.

Since I've always been so vital, John feels I will bounce back readily. He prefers to treat me with a natural immune-support protocol of powerful herbs and homeopathy versus an antibiotic. I get a shot of colloidal silver and some supplies, and crawl back home to bed. Again, I have to cancel another few days of clients, but I figure by next week I should be fine.

John leaves for a two-week vacation on Friday. By the weekend I can't stand up without the room spinning. My head is awash in a foggy, cottony heaviness. My eyelids feel like sandbags are dragging them down. All my limbs still ache and the weakness is extreme. It's frightening for me to feel so depleted in one week's time. His on-call doctor can't see me until next week. I start the ten-day backup prescription of amoxicillin John has left on call for me at the pharmacy.

"This will pull me out of it for sure," I mutter through the stupor.

A week later, July 4 comes and I'm still a mess. The world is some sort of hazy place with me locked in a chamber of gauze. I've never felt so out of sorts. I call my usual GP/gynecologist, since John is still away. She calls me back and I relay the entire situation to her on the phone. Given the profound exhaustion and no response to the antibiotic, Nora thinks perhaps it's walking pneumonia.

"Come in and see my associate physician, Dr. Cummings," she says. "I'm booked solid this week. I can slip you in with him."

Joel takes me in. I get a chest X-ray, they shoot me up with a bazooka antibiotic, and I go home to collapse back into bed. It could take six weeks to heal, I've been told. Something feels intuitively not right about this walking pneumonia diagnosis. I've never had a bacterial infection in my life, other than the common-variety female bladder infection. My respiratory and lymph systems have essentially been impenetrable. I have a strange itchy rash on my chest, violent headaches, roiling gut upset, and no cough. Plus, my heart takes off in irregular rhythms now and then. Anxiety and panic are popping up, and my neck hurts a lot.

Strangely, too, the left side of my face has numb sensations and a droopy feeling when I talk. It's like a mild Bell's palsy. As a natural health practitioner, I know a little too much—enough to make me worry excessively at times.

A few days later, I go back to Nora's office. More of the killer antibiotic is shot into my gluteus muscle. Back home, I need help up the stairs because I'm so weak. This illness is too overwhelming to believe.

"I feel so horribly sick, Joel," I whimper. "Pneumonia is just awful."

He encourages me to relax. "You'll be well again soon, Kim. Try to be patient."

Meanwhile, all hell breaks loose in the household. Laundry, dishes, and toys are strewn haphazardly. Joel's work piles up. My three-year-old son can't understand why Mommy is stuck in bed, unable to get up and play. I'm so weak I need help just showering. Joel must steer me to the bathroom and shampoo my hair while I hold onto the shower curtain bar. Then I'm wiped out for another two hours and can't move a muscle in bed. It's exhausting just to breathe. The world spins. I feel strangely frightened.

Perfect summer days sail by outside my bedroom window. I peer out through the fluttering cotton sheers, staring at the weeds accumulating in my gardens, watching the foxglove grow, my meadow rue bloom, and the bee balm gather the tender, ruby-throated hummingbirds. Church people cook some meals for us, and the kindly elderly minister pays me a call. It's an enormous effort to sit on the deck with him for twenty minutes. In all honesty, it's tiring just to hold my head up.

In the midst of this drama, our very capable and treasured babysitter quits. It's like a shipwreck. I can't function. Joel travels constantly with his work. In fact, he's off to Bruges, Belgium, in a week. Neither of us have family in the area. They're all in Florida and New York. By now I'm crying a lot. It's almost unfathomable to me that I am so sick I can't even make a sandwich. A good day is when I can make it down the stairs for a meal. I lay in wait for my healing. Others reassure me that it will come, but it seems to be taking forever. I ask a colleague in Vermont to take over my clients. Thankfully, he does. My world is falling away from me. I'm losing control of any and all things I know. I feel horrified and traumatized.

When Joel must fly to Chicago on business for three days, my dad comes to stay with Eli and me. George is not used to toddlers, but somehow we do okay. Lying limp in bed, my dad giving me a pep talk, a lightbulb notion clicks within me: perhaps we should hire an au pair to live with us. That would be better than trying to hire another rotating local sitter.

When Joel returns, we start the process with an established agency in Boston, which is easier said than done. It all takes time. Bringing over a girl from Europe will take us a minimum of eight weeks. By then, I will be well—theoretically. Joel and I decide to go for it anyway. It's more affordable than local help. Plus, with our demanding careers, we need reliable care for Eli. As believers in homespun footing for young children, we don't want to traverse the day care route. We are struggling on all fronts by now.

In short order Joel leaves again for a solid week. I'm a sobbing mess. How will I ever handle an energetic, imploring three-year-old when I can't even care for myself?

I call my stalwart aunt in Florida. "SOS! I need help!"

Aunt Connie flies in. She patches things together for me: cooking, running errands, playing with Eli, making me believe I'll get well. She does a fine job.

"You're a Makris, don't forget," Connie proclaims. "Your forebears all lived into their nineties. We're tough. So are you. You know how to heal. It'll just take some time. Really, Kim," she resolutely pronounces, "it will all pass." Then she gets back to work scrubbing the dishes clean.

I lie on the sofa, lost in a tepid fog. Sitting up to eat I feel like an amoeba. Cutting my meat is an effort. They prop me up on the chaise lounge on a sunny July day. I watch Eli playing freely in the glade of cinnamon ferns. There he stands in the vivid brocade, only the tips of his shiny hair and glittering eyes cresting above the greenery. Echo proudly attempts to "herd" the chickens, showing me how capable she is. I hear our borrowed summertime sheep bleating in the distance, bells tinkling as they wander. Joel is due home tonight. I look forward to his sturdy presence. He makes me feel safe. Maybe I'll feel less worn when he arrives. I conjure up images of me improving, dancing in the moonlight with my handsome husband.

Somehow I get through the week. But the stress bearing down on me is enormous. My confidence is totally shot. Fear grips my every breath. Panic attacks strike in the middle of the night now. I wake Joel, my heart throbbing, my chest gripped in a vise.

"Help me," I beg. "Hold me. I'm scared."

"You'll be okay, Kim," he soothes as he pulls me to his chest. "Take some deep breaths."

My not getting well is not my only fear. I don't know how to cope with being so dependent on others. It's not my forte. I've always been so fearless and capable. I don't feel like I'm making any progress. My trusted homeopathic remedies are the only things that boost me along, though very moderately. I need something to hold on to. I imagine myself healthy and vital, climbing my favorite spruce-trimmed peak, laughing at a party, working at my office. I know positive imagery does wonders. Now, it merely pads the walls of my frantic mind.

Time limps along. As we round the four-week mark, Joel and Eli go to collect Sarah at camp. I'm alone at home, wasted. It's a time of crushing solitude, insecurity, and ominous foreboding. Is this that towering storm image I gleaned while sitting by Wyeth's body? My beloved border collie lies for hours at my bedside. She senses my sadness and won't let down her watch. Shaking and emptied, I break my steadfast No Dog Allowed rule and permit Echo to sleep in my room. She sits patiently with me, my flaccid arm draped down from the bedside, my hand stroking her ebony fur. We await the au pair from Poland.

"Help will come," I whisper. "Soon."

Raven Calls

The summer continues to drone along at a halting pace. Still reeling from the quake of my derailment, the first weekend in August I decide to go stay at a friend's house. Having been stranded at home for a treacherously long seven weeks, I'm gripped by a stifling cabin fever. Joel and I agree that it might do my spirits good to see a few walls different from my own. Charlene has been a dear friend for many years. In fact, we worked together at the same clinic on my arrival to New England nine years ago. We are like family, really, close in heart and spirit. With grown children and living alone, Charlene welcomes me with open arms. A friend for the weekend is a pleasurable change in her routine.

I slip into the soft bedsheets of her third floor bedroom, listening to the wind whisper in her towering white pines. The north woods are lush and strongly scented at summer's height. As I settle under my covers in the lavender twilight, I can't help noticing the persistent cawing of ravens perched high in the pine boughs. On and on they chatter amongst themselves as I drift benignly to sleep.

A heavy dream draws me into endless corridors and a confusing labyrinth of minotaur-like chases. I'm trying to run and escape the clutches of a looming dark force at my heels. A raven's voice guides me through the darkness and low-ceilinged crawlways. Instinctively, I follow its rasping call. "The call of death binds you," he caws. Suddenly, after a quick turn at the stoney corner, I'm out, into the sun and onto a dewy, green lawn. I look up to see the bright, shimmering, coal-dark eyes of an ebony-feathered raven laughing with me, in my abrupt burst into freedom and safety. I wake from my dream, thinking of the raven. A trickster, a clever one, its knowing glance and laughing caw heralds a way out of my misery. I slip back into sleep again.

I awaken in the morning quietly and somehow less laden by oppressive fatigue. By midmorning, after resting on Charlene's outside chaise lounge, I actually shock myself and take a moderate walk down and back her long dirt driveway. I sense I'm on the mend. The doctors were right; it would take about six weeks to recover. I'm hopeful that this "walking pneumonia" is passing, again glimpsing the laughing raven in my mind's eye.

The rest of August I slowly advance in strength, though not greatly in stamina. I'm vertical a lot more, able to cook a meal now and then, and amazingly I can empty the dishwasher. As August stretches into September, we take our annual trip to a family camp in Vermont. I'm much less physical than in years past. In fact, I notice this weird fullness and pain in my left side, near my ribs and spleen, when swimming or jumping. Even when laughing too hard, it hurts. But the time spent outside is just gorgeous. I feel fed by the beauty of the outdoors.

A few short days after we return, Sarah starts middle school, while Eli and I await our au pair. I begin to wonder if family camp was too much for me, as my energy does not pick up much, now ten weeks after becoming ill. I feel anxious and stressed when my husband leaves for a workweek in Europe. Driving to town for errands has felt draining to me, and vicious migraines can still hit me by surprise. This vulnerability ripples striations of tentative insecurity through me. On many days I feel as if I walk on newborn Bambi-like legs. Eli and I survive on our own, though I'm much more worn and weary when Joel comes home.

"The au pair should help buffer me some," I try to reassure him.

"I'm certain she will," he encourages, tension reflected in his taut smile. Joel is trying hard to help me and cope with the stress of this unexpected illness. Will he really be able to handle it all, as he is so entrenched in his fast-paced career and need for daily trifles managed to the nth degree? Joel has always valued me as a wife for being, as he says in Yiddish, a mensch, a woman who can take care of herself. I'm nothing like that now. I'm weak and needy, barely able to manage a few days on my own.

I think of that first night I met Joel. It was only the second blind date of my life, the first having been at a fraternity rush party in college. I didn't know exactly how I felt about this, other than basically cooperating with a friend's best intentions. Rene coaxed me along, pledging that Joel was sweet and kind and broken up over having been left by his first wife.

"Joel will really appreciate your fun-loving spirit," she promised. "Plus, you're both from New York. You'll be good for him."

I trusted Rene's judgment, as she had a stellar husband and deeply loving marriage to show for it.

Oh, well, I thought, *I'll give it a whirl. One date is not a big deal.* "Nothing ventured, nothing gained" was my life motto anyway. But then again that cavalier, risk-taking attitude was how I had ended up married to my megalomaniac former husband, our engagement pledged on a whim one month into a high-flying courtship.

Joel called to invite me out before I could change my mind. He sounded nice enough on the phone: intelligent, friendly, even a mutual interest in blues music. Initially, Joel suggested that we go out to dinner, but then he called back to rearrange, saying that he would cook for me and I should come to his home. Hesitant at first, as per my forever careful mother's warning never to be alone with a stranger, I finally figured it was safe enough, as so many community acquaintances knew Joel Bendhem as a respected businessman and a self-confident, likable "good guy."

I stopped for flowers on the way to Joel's home in the late summer of 1994. My favorite blue summer dress, with its dainty print and sweetheart neckline, made me feel girlishly pretty. It was a glorious August evening, with the first kiss of autumn's chill in the air. I felt a sudden whip of butterflies in my stomach as I pulled into his driveway.

What am I doing? I thought. *I have no clue who this man is!*

But suddenly, I was parking in front of a red-shingled saltbox home in the slightly darkened lee of a hillside backdrop, with a well-maintained lawn and comfortable ambience. The moss-pocked brick walkway felt slippery and bumpy under my feet as I anxiously stepped up to the door, which swung open, showcasing a tall, dark-haired man who, thankfully, showed the gift of depth in his eyes. He smiled. We exchanged greetings and the flowers, and coltishly I stepped inside.

I could see sliced avocado with crackers and a bottle of Merlot awaiting me on the kitchen counter. We either had the same taste in appetizers or Joel had done some homework on me. The friendly small talk sashayed between us. He was easy to chat with, open, engaging, and rather rakishly charming. We talked about our New York ethnic up-bringings over a well-prepared meal on his screened-in back porch. I liked him. It wasn't a drop-to-your-knees kind of attraction, but the comfort level and rapport were pleasant enough.

Decent guy, I surmised. *Not bad for a blind date.*

Before long, though, Joel was in tears, sharing the story of his mar-riage's collapse and the pressures of being a part-time single father to a four-year-old daughter. With all my years of experience counseling oth-ers through their woes, I was an easy shoulder to cry on.

"It's all right, Joel, really," I consoled. "I understand pain. Don't worry about crying."

I tried to lighten the scene by suggesting a walk in his brim-ming yard.

The poolside garden was cheerful and laden with crimson dahlias, thriving clumps of phlox, and trailing clematis. The dying sun's red-dened rays cast a poignant painter's light on the tops of the tallest plants. In fact, they seemed to glow in their collective beauty. What struck my eye, however, was an enormous, fully blooming bleeding heart plant, tucked over on the far side of the pool shed. Gingerly, I picked up one of its elegant stalks of exquisite red-and-white miniature hearts. They dangled in a graceful string as I drew them close for a glimpse at their delicate beauty.

"Joel," I asked, "why is this blooming now, in August instead of May?"

"I don't know. It started to bloom according to its normal cycle and then just never stopped," he told me. For some reason, this prolific plant left me with an unexpected feeling of foreboding. As we veered back indoors, I felt a ghostly shiver shimmy down my spine. I turned to look at Joel, but he appeared strong, composed; it was a reassuring sign.

The night ended on a rather upbeat note, me filling Joel in on details of the beautiful new home that I would be closing on the next day and he telling me about his upcoming business trip to New York. I ambled out to the car, crystal starlight twinkling brightly through the pines, on a buzzy wave of optimism about this pleasant evening. As I turned on the engine, the radio station streamed outward with a song from my childhood, so rarely played anymore: "Someday My Prince Will Come." I couldn't help but wonder.

Lying here, half-mast and struggling, I'm gripped with the fear that I'll never get better. My guilty feelings over being ill gnaw an ulcerous worry within. I tremble, gazing at the lovely world of beauty beckoning outside my bedroom window. That bleeding heart appears in my mind's eye. Why can't I recover? I'm still not back seeing clients.

Shockingly, our long-awaited help from Poland ends up being a two-week travesty of domino-like stressful events. With Hannah's first step out of the car onto our welcoming, balloon-garbed front porch, she bursts into tears.

"It's not a city!" she bemoans.

"We told you we live in the country," I reply, as optimistically as I can. I am taken aback, though.

Nothing goes well. Hannah sits and stares at our three-year-old son. She does not know how to play with a toddler. Her driving skills are atrocious and she is afraid to cook any meals. Hannah is MIA for over six hours when attempting to go to an au pair agency meeting forty-five minutes away. The police pick her up swaying over the yellow road line in Maine! The final straw comes two weeks later, when Hannah is backing up the ten-year-old Chevy Astro van we purchased for her. As I glance out the living room window, my heart arrests then rockets off the maps, as Hannah blazes backward in the drive, careening the tank-like vehicle straight into the woods directly at an enormous oak. Eli is a passenger, blessedly strapped into his car seat. He is unscathed.

I have had enough. The agency ships Hannah off to a family of seven in Chicago. Meanwhile my nerves are shot and my health rapidly declines. In fact, it's worse than in the summer: my limbs barely hold me up, my bowels are a mess, and migraines last for three solid days at a time.

"I'm sicker than ever," I wail to my sympathetic physician in early October. "I've never felt so weak in my entire life. Check me for everything!"

Nora examines me and draws numerous vials of blood, then Charlene transports me back home, tucking me once again into bed. I'm spent, weak as a newborn kitten. Fear, confusion, and a sense of deep, gaping despair overwhelm my reason as my mind reels with possible diagnoses. Finally, Nora calls with test results.

"There's good news and bad, Kim," she says.

It isn't cancer or lupus or anything so severe, but Nora tells me that I have a case of Epstein-Barr virus.

"I have mono?" I ask. "What about the pneumonia?"

"Sort of, but not exactly," she explains. "You have an outbreak or reactivation of an older case of mononucleosis. Did you have it when you were younger, in your teens or twenties?"

I tell her that I'm not sure. "Maybe in 1983, right after my first wedding. I was so weak and breathlessly sick on our honeymoon that my husband had to carry me up and down the Spanish Steps in Rome. Romantic, huh?"

Nora agrees that that may have been the initial infection and that, now, the walking pneumonia has worn me down and left me vulnerable to a recurring outbreak.

"It's in the same family as herpes," she tells me, "so when your system becomes stressed or weak, the Epstein-Barr virus can have a breakout."

I have helped many clients with Epstein-Barr over the years, so I know all about it. EBV can be a culprit behind chronic fatigue syndrome, and I definitely don't want to go there.

"Okay, at least I have an idea of what to address now. My homeopathic remedies should help me make it dormant again," I glumly reply.

Nora wants me on another six weeks of bed rest, with no stress and lots of sleep. "Drink lots of fluids, too," she says, confident that I'll be able to handle my own recovery process.

I'm not so sure. Joel travels so much, and I don't know how I'm going to manage myself and the kids in this condition. It's all too much for me. And the more sickening news is the au pair agency can't find us a replacement girl until the new year!

"Please," I beg, "I'm so ill! Can't you find us another girl?"

The agency tells me that our family is difficult to place with our remote country location, which seems just silly to me. Our charming town is a mere five miles away.

"See if you can make a miracle happen," I plead.

Down I slide into many long months of dreary oblivion, days spent in what feels like the worst jet lag of my life. Our home life is shattering around me. Everyone suffers when a mother is stricken ill. It's as if the heart of the family is broken. All the softness, the nurturance, the tending of everyone's needs whirl down the drain. Daily chores, laundry, groceries, muddy shoes, bills all fall into disarray. School projects, childhood boo-boos, Halloween costumes swirl around us in a maelstrom of disharmony. Joel pinch-hits constantly, juggling meals and shampoos, lists ad infinitum.

"Mommy can't do that right now, she's resting," he repeats all too often.

Tiptoed footsteps, dinner on TV trays in our bedroom, and sticky jamprints on the walls filter through my haze of frustration and plummeting spirits. Joel must work to keep our income stable. My cleaning woman arrives one Tuesday and is horrified to find me home alone with Eli, Joel in Europe, and me ashen on the sofa, too dizzy to make it up the stairs. She calls her home, collects her daughter, and selflessly stays with me another three days until my husband returns. I can't function. *How can my entire world be collapsing on me?*

Finally, as the snow piles up and the days darken to a smoky gray at best, we get word that an au pair is arriving for us from the Czech Republic at the first of the year. Relief is in sight! Quiet tears of self-pity stain my pillow; I try to hold on to my sensibilities.

Relief

Sophie arrives to us on a sterling winter's day, sunshine filling the sky on the heels of last night's fresh snowfall. This time, the greeting goes much more smoothly. With my three memorized Czech words, we welcome a kind and thoughtful young woman into our family. Sophie is intelligent, gentle, patient, and very good with children. She has a younger brother, nine years her junior. We help Sophie get settled into her room. She has the large converted office/playroom space above the garage. Two huge plate-glass windows overlook the yard and neighbors. A high cathedral ceiling, her own TV and stereo, plus a sofa area, desk, and separate thermostat make this spot private from our family, yet cheery and comfortable for Sophie.

Within a week's time we navigate the language barrier together, a dictionary and sign language tipping each of us into giggling spells. The feeling is much more convivial and warm with Sophie than it had been with Hannah. She is tall and strong, immediately hoisting Eli high above her shoulders in airplane spins. Sophie skis and appreciates the natural beauty of our environment. Before long she is at the local mountain with Joel and the kids, swooshing down the slopes, laughing in her sunny way. Eli and Sarah take to her instantly. Board games, Play-Doh, and indoor forts made of bedsheets stretch through the living room. An enormous weight lifts from my shoulders.

It takes a bit of time to teach Sophie how to grocery shop for our particular foodstuffs in a long-aisled A&P, which is so different from her small market at home. But soon she masters that, as well as our laundry machines and other modern household conveniences. Most of the twenty-one-year-olds we know are off to college, and I worry that Sophie will be lonely without peers. Through a friend of mine we get word of two young Czech men who live locally and work at a facility for the handicapped. She is too reserved ever to dream of calling these men on her own, so I arrange for Joel to escort Sophie to our local pub to meet up with her compatriots. All goes swimmingly. The guys are fun and zany. Best of all, however, is that at the monthly regional au pair dinner, Sophie finds another Czech au pair to hang out with. Before long Nika is at our home for weekends. The two are a whirlwind of hairstyles, jewelry, and chatter. Their youthful energy is delightful.

By February I'm still a weak, foggy mess, though. Sophie has helped bring order back to our household, but my health is really not any different. Tensions run high between me and Joel. The romance and affection in our relationship have been replaced with inadequacies and building resentments. Spats break out over mundane events. I become impatient and snappish, having been cooped up for almost eight months. Trying to accept being so out of control is insanely difficult. I long for happier times.

Lying on the sofa in my now familiar horizontal pose, I study the cheerful gathering of framed photographs dotting our walls and tables. Merry smiles and brilliant love gaze back at me. I become entranced with a marvelous shot of Joel and me, arms encircled and hearts erupting, standing along the river Seine, the grand Eiffel Tower in the backdrop. Immediately, I'm thrown backward in time to the heady days of our celestial courtship when this picture was taken.

In 1994, as I settled into my new home, nestled deep in the untrampled New Hampshire woods, Joel wooed me in a courtship of sweeping romantic proportions. I felt as if we were flying through the starry nights and sun-splattered days in a state of perpetual ecstasy. Every breath I took was filled with a madly growing love for this man of keen mind, witty humor, and deeply rooted passions. We were a pair of firebursts, fueling each other's purpose and desires.

As the burnished twilight of autumn descended, Joel and I spent days and nights soaking in one another, weaving together in the way only destiny can lay its spell. Late nights over wine and savories, hikes in the crinkling amber woods, long canoe paddles on mirrored waters, and lazy Sundays entwined together knitted our bond.

"I've never seen you so caught up in a man before," my friend Lila said to me one day on the car ride back from shopping. "You must be really crazy about him."

She was right; I loved him wildly. It felt like kismet with Joel. I had met my match, a man who could meet me square-on. We were both firstborns, ambitious, hardworking, and smart. We knew how to push the envelope of life, yet not go too far over the edge. Family oriented and planted in a love of the outdoors, we shared many interests and tastes, and our mutual orientation toward world cultures and inner growth enlivened the brew.

Though my dear mother was slipping away into the grip of cancer, my heart was buoyed by the grand love erupting between Joel and me. Love notes fluttering under my windshield wiper and weekends whisked away to snow-clad inns marked our affair with an aura of magic. Joel and I claimed our love for one another to be of legendary proportions. Anthony and Cleopatra, Romeo and Juliet—these were our kindred spirits.

Joel brought me along on a springtime work trip to Europe. The medieval graces of Bruges held me in wonder, while the mysterious hauntings of Normandy's ancient chateaus and sweeping poppy fields wooed my artistic spirit from hiding. By the time Joel and I arrived in Paris, I recognized that my heart was bound to his.

Back home in my New Hampshire forest, Joel's soft-spoken, five-year-old daughter, Sarah, and I found a quiet kinship together, playing dress-up and cooking in the kitchen. We laughed ourselves silly one rain-damp afternoon as Echo panicked at being adorned with two-foot-tall, glitter-encrusted fairy wings. Sarah liked my voice. "It's so soft. It's like a bell," she said. I loved her angel-fine sensitivity. I learned that Joel wanted more children, and a Thumbelina dose of pleasure warmed my heart, urging my already straining biological clock to tick even louder.

Joel and I found our perfected symmetry in the silken waters of Tulum, Mexico. Under the shadow of the ancient Temple of the Winds he asked me to marry. And so we were wed on the snow-dressed eve of the winter's solstice 1996, surrounded by seventy-five close friends and family, including the yet-unborn life that grew inside me. The unique ceremony combined our faiths and traditions, sentiments and dreams. The restored historical barn glowed with candlelight, and a tiger-orange fire roared in the enormous fireplace. Amidst festoons of fragrant greens and the benevolence of surrounding joy, I had never felt so happy and hopeful.

In the muddy, earthen days of April, we welcomed our beautiful son into the world. Our family was now perfectly formed with four foundational corners. Eli cried and cooed, spit up and smiled. New motherhood bathed me in contentment. The days blended into nights and months stretched into years. We were as one.

But now I feel the misery of these months of illness. Oh, how I resent the ugliness of this past year. There's so much to be grateful for, in spite of the losses. I need to accept this process and become more patient with myself, my body, and my husband. But such things are often easier said than done. I'm miserable trapped in the house, unable to work and care for all that I love, my family and practice included. I feel tremendous sorrow at having let my clients down, not being there to care for them. I know they do not feel as aligned with my replacement homeopath as they did with me. Joel is stretched beyond his capacity. Eli is confused. Sarah is coping as best she can. How I hate this plummet of depression and loss. I hold on to my hopes and dreams in order to cope.

Winter looms large.

School vacation week in late February marks our annual pilgrimage to visit family in south Florida. Joel and I fortunately both have our immediate relations living there. This year my friend Charlene and I leave a week early, figuring the extra warmth and sea bathing should be restorative for me. The journey down the coast feels abysmal, however. Trying to walk between the terminal gates on our plane transfer in Philadelphia is overwhelming. Two times we need to stop and let me sit down to rest. My limbs are quaky, my head spinning, but we finally arrive in Fort Lauderdale with me in one piece.

We stay at my father's magnificent condo, high in the sky and situated on a stunning stretch of eggshell-white beachfront. I soak in the sun like a sponge. On the first dip in the pool all I can muster is a floating-style swim to one end and back. By the time Joel and the troops arrive a full week later, I have steadily worked up to ten lengths. He tells me that I look scrumptious with my cocoa-brown suntan.

"I have never seen such colors," Sophie tells me. "The sea is like a dream."

And it is. In totality, I spend four glorious weeks at my father's. It does all of us a world of good. Although I'm still not a hundred percent, I feel better than I have since before I got ill nine months ago. We even manage a few outings to the Science Museum and Monkey Jungle. It appears the vitamin D, ocean salts, and rest have knocked out the virus. Victory! Eventually, my time in the sun comes to a close. We journey northward, back home to the soppy-wet snowfalls of spring.

Northbound

Returning to our snug home and comely town I note a new attitude within. I'm relieved to be feeling stronger, plus the marital bruises appear to be eased by our Floridian vacation. Summertime and good weather are right around the corner, heralding the best months of life in our region. I'm thinking it is time I get back to work, maybe even just a couple of days per week. I miss my clients and office, plus the great sense of fulfillment homeopathy gives me. I decide to check in with my physician, Nora, before booking appointments. Unfortunately, my blood work brings us bad news.

"The Epstein-Barr virus is still active, Kim. You're out of the acute infection, but still in a secondary phase, which we call convalescence. It hasn't gotten to the dormant phase yet."

My heart drops low. "I feel so much better," I tell her. "I was hoping to get back to work."

But she is adamant that it is not yet time for me to resume that level of activity. "We need to see these titres at the post-infection stage," Nora tells me. "Rest up some more. Take some gentle walks outdoors and let's recheck you again in six weeks. Don't push yourself so hard. The clients are in good hands. They can wait a little longer."

I nod in sullen compliance.

On the way back to the house I decide to stop at my office just to soak in its ambience. I'll pick up my mail and say hi to my friends in the neighboring suites. Everything looks just the same as before as I sit in the tall-back swivel desk chair, surveying the room. The Caribbean floral-print sofa is vibrant and happy looking. My photos and books are all in their exact spots. I gaze out the numerous sunny windows upon our picturesque New England town, the slate roofs shining in the softened March air and the proud white church steeple stretching above the scene in timeless watch. All seems content. Inside me, however, much churns. How I long to be back here working, my day chock-full with clients, the phone ringing, children banging toys around in the play area.

I've spent nine years lovingly tending to this practice. I'm devoted to this work, my newspaper health column, and the people I help. Sitting here in solitude I reflect on all the hard work I have put into this career and life. I think back to my arrival here, in the beginning.

In my aged Jeep, with a mere $250, two boxes, and a daring love of adventure bolstering my spirit, I left my Long Island North Shore upbringing behind and headed to New Hampshire to redesign my life. I was fleeing an imploding and dangerous marriage, but my chic mother was aghast at my move to rural New England.

"How will you survive in the cold and isolation, Kim? This just goes against my grain," Patricia beseeched.

"It is not that different from our summers in Vermont, Mother," I countered. "It's lovely. Have Dad drive you up next month when the leaves change so you can see for yourself."

"Oh, darling, summers were quaint. Winters will be foreboding. Keep yourself safe and warm," she said, stuffing a box of fleece everything into my car—jacket, hat, mittens, blanket included. "Drive safely and call us when you get there!"

She waved good-bye against the backdrop of her estate house, the image receding in my rearview mirror. A lump formed in my throat as I darted down the drive.

A solar-designed holistic health center awaited me in September 1991, offering a career amongst like-minded practitioners. This was a rare opportunity to bring homeopathic medicine back into America's life, out of the closet in which it had lain dormant for five decades.

I sensed that this was a time and place where I could call my own shots and bring the best of my skills to others.

My new residence was an airy A-frame rented home, cresting a pristine highland lake. I settled into the woods that autumn with the conscious intention to live a simpler life, close to the land. While cities and chaos made me feel hurried and blurry, I was centered and calm deep in the mysterious woods, with its musky smells and changing beauty.

I adapted immediately to my new environs, hiking and horseback riding with newfound friends. The frosty air of autumn filled my lungs with a rich blend of power, excitement, and fancy for this startling new beginning. Come winter I found myself donning graying high school ice skates and gliding freely across the glassy, expansive frozen lake at my driveway's threshold. My spirit soared as I traced the edges of the cloaked shoreline, heaving in armloads of snowy splendor. Here I was, alone in the north woods, without my family or any security, carving more into the ice than a figure eight. I carved the foundation for my new life.

It was a bold move to come to an unknown land, without any guarantee of success, but I had confidence that I could build a sustainable homeopathic practice while helping others with my knowledge. Hard work and courage were bred deeply in the marrow of my paternal family's bloodline. Raised from the hardiest of Grecian stock, we are a strong and willful clan, shying away from nothing much. Like my daring and enormously powerful father before me, I believed I could count on my vigorous constitution and boundless energy to achieve my dreams. After all, my father was the best of teachers, planting the message of hope and possibility within me since childhood.

"The backyard is not your playground," he told me again and again. "The neighborhood is not your playground, nor is the state of New York. The entire world is yours, Kim! Work hard and you can be anything you want to be in this lifetime. There are no limits." His inspiration has been my bedrock of possibilities.

I did work hard over the ensuing years at the clinic and teaching homeopathic classes. Gentleness and empathic understanding were my trademarks as a healer. A frontier spirit at heart, I developed many professional alliances within the conventional medical arena. Before long,

I was writing a popular health column in a regional newspaper. It all flowed effortlessly and prodigiously.

When it came time to purchase a home of my own, three years after my move north, I gravitated to a unique dwelling centered in the forest. Putting down some firm roots was in order, as I had created a successful homeopathic practice in a region of hale Yankees and independent thinkers.

The home I found, where we still live, is a simple Cape best described as a work of art. A post-and-beam construction, made of solid oak and cherry, each beam is held together by hand-hewn wooden pegs in an elaborate jigsaw puzzle design. With open cathedral ceilings upstairs, it's like looking into the hull of an old wooden-masted schooner, ribs and planking holding fast. Here we feel cozy and secure.

Situated on the back roads at the outskirts of our idyllic town of Greenvale, it all feels storybook lovely. Greenvale is a thriving New England town filled with wholesome goodness, artistic flare, and a solid measure of steady composure. It's a family place, ordered and simple in its no-fuss lifestyle. Our quintessential postcard downtown harbors just about one of everything. Just enough to get by on: one stationery store, one traffic light, an old-fashioned hundred-seat cinema, and a family-owned corner market. We also proudly boast a splendid summer stock theater, and many fine trails to hike. Little League baseball, catching pollywogs in tranquil ponds, and the annual Fourth of July fireworks bonanza seal in the Norman Rockwell charm.

Our town is wholesome and friendly. It does, however, lack that tweak of pizzazz that some need to keep the pulses going and avoid lapsing into "coma-like" status, as my continental, octane-fueled father complains.

"I don't know how you can survive up there, Kim. Half the people are embalmed. Do they have a pulse?" George asks me, in his typical sardonic humor.

I laugh it off and reply, "It's a good town, Daddy. It's a great place to raise kids. If you like the outdoors you couldn't ask for more. Look at the beauty, plus the skiing and hiking."

"Yeah, yeah. That's true about the family environment, but Jesus, you can't even get a good kaiser roll up there!" he grumbles and jests simultaneously.

"Point taken," I say. "I happen to like it here, though, you know. The easier pace suits me. I'm not as impervious as you to the hell-bent tempo of New York and the maniac drivers."

"The drivers really are a disaster, aren't they? I take my life in my hands every day on that goddamn L.I.E! Well, as long as you're happy, honey. That's what counts."

So it goes with my family's perpetual confusion over my move to the country. He's right, but somehow that doesn't seem to matter to me. Tramping through six months of the year in L. L. Bean boots and heavy woolen sweaters did certainly wean the swanky silkens and designer suits out of my repertoire. Way back in the dusty reaches of my closet, a few choice frocks lie in wait for the occasional benefit dinner dance or a sojourn home to see the family in New York. But slowly, over the years, New Hampshire has managed to spin the fluff out of me—kitten heels, tulle, and beads included. Sturdy, dependable, and comfortable are words that I have come to value across the board—clothing, vehicles, and men included.

Eventually, I moved from the clinic into private practice with a holistically minded MD, Dr. John Miller.

Joel and I have woven together a lifestyle of conscious healthful living: organic gardening, simple pleasures, family time, and armfuls of friends surrounding us. We have been graced.

Now I worry that I'm on the verge of losing my career. Determined to quell this EBV, I pull out my homeopathic books, cross-reference symptoms and remedies, and settle upon one I believe will help me. I'm determined to be well!

Painting

Alittle bit of magic enters my life a month later. Since childhood I have yearned to learn how to paint properly. Rainy days and idle hours I would often sketch, musing and passing the time, with my long braids stretched down my arms, pencil and pad in hand. Art class was just okay at my school and my mother was not much of a driver, uninterested in toting me off to private painting lessons, as much as I begged her.

"You can teach yourself to paint, Kim," Patricia always said. "You know I hate to drive far"—which meant anything more than about ten minutes from our home. So Mother got me some watercolors and I experimented with the lazy drift of colors and shapes meandering across the linen paper, creating orbs and elves, trees and animals, at the feather tip of the sable brush.

Now, decades later, with my homeopathic prescription boosting my vitality, I decide to sign up for a still-life class at a local art school. I figure it will be good for my spirits after such an arduous winter. The first day of class is like a scene out of *I Love Lucy* as I stand there in a room full of artists, confused even over how to erect the easel. The instructor warbles on about mixing thallos and cadmiums and I am completely perplexed about what to do with these paint-laden, messy brushes. My palette is a muddy mix of sticky paint, the canvas looks more abstract than real, and I'm clearly the blundering neophyte amongst the wizards of color and glory, deftly stroking out petals and vases with ease and grace before my very eyes. Before long, I'm woozy from the vapors and smeared in paint. The remarkable thing is that I love it!

The buttery paint moves sensuously beneath my brush. It's an alchemy of sorts to transfer the flowers and apples from the tabletop to the canvas. Both fun and a challenge, oil painting is a winning combination for me. I'm addicted, eagerly awaiting my weekly class, which is incentive enough to haul my wilted spirit out of the house and away from malingering malaise. By class three I'm on fire, prancing in the front door with my first completed painting, proud as a peacock.

When the plein-air landscape class rolls around in June, I'm unstoppable. Painting out of doors in the elements inspires me in huge ways. I feel a rush of ecstasy roll through me with the sunlight and wind cavorting around me and the environs. A whole new language and world is opening to me through paint. I'm in awe, and it's beautiful.

Every decent day I leave Eli with Sophie and dash out the door to a new locale, painting scenes of the region in a delirious passion of creativity. I use Sarah's music stand for an easel and my kitchen apron as a smock. Although I must be quite a sight, I am blooming in the sheer delight of the discovery that I can paint, and pretty darn well, at that. People start purchasing my little vignettes, while friends marvel at this hidden talent bursting forth from me in a radiant spray. All I can do is laugh and swim in the euphoria of my adventure. It's a gift, I know. The plentiful time in the outdoors, plus the creative expression, is healing to me.

With a reclaimed enthusiasm for life, I actually feel well enough to take a camping trip with Joel and the kids. We smile and play together and feel like a family again.

As September enters, with pristine light and still afternoons, I sense a wholeness and solidity in me. What a godsend, I think, as we slip into the season of mystical change. Autumn leaves swirl in brilliant hues of orange and red, kaleidoscoping in an ecstatic finale of beauty, before the bitter crunch of winter wraps us tight. I try to capture it all on my canvases. And yes, I begin to see a few former clients in my office.

Home Fires

In the dimming light of November, treetops shimmy barren and stark during a cold afternoon's rainfall. Only the intrepid beeches hold the last traces of leaves, a mustard-brown spangle of jewelry amid the other soldier-straight trunks of the forest. I throw more logs into the woodstove to fend off the chill. The radiant heat of our able Vermont Castings keeps us cozy and warm, as shoe-sized puddles pool outside our glass-paned back door. Glimpsing a stray yellow Tonka truck under the lofty hemlock and some random balls scattered about where the children left them last, I chink a mental note to remind Sarah and Eli to bring them in tonight, as snow is likely any day now.

Our country home rests high on a granite ridge, nestled within the thick forest and snaking, ancient stone walls of long-gone homesteads. It's a woodland wonder, abundant with deer, owls, and even a mama bear. With snow patches still banking the driveway and the north face of the buildings, on softening March mornings we find her big, broad paw prints on either side of the snapped bird feeder. *Is that why Echo barked so furiously in the night?*

Life in the woods requires an adventurous spirit and an appreciation for the force of the elements, plus a good, strong backbone. My senses are nourished endlessly by this closely entwined relationship to nature. The sound of a brazen winter wind howling down the smoking chimney, setting the air plate on the woodstove into a flap, stirs a strain of excitement in my blood. The April chirrupings of mating peepers soothe us to sleep in evening chorus. It's captivating to see an elusive, sleek, brown mink silently undulating along the tumbling stone wall out back or, even more regularly, to hear the chilling howls and plaintive wails of a coyote pack breaking the stillness of a deep winter's night.

As I close the henhouse door tight, tugging the rusty-hinged wood across crunching snow, I look up into the rich, velvet-black sky to see the luminescent twinkle of a million magical stars gleaming back at me. I never tire of that glance upward into the majesty of the heavens showering from above. That overpowering sense of awe and beauty reminds me why I moved up to these backwood hills in the first place.

My husband and I live a life close to the land, tending to our home fires and children with care and devotion. We rake heaving mounds of snow off the roof in winter, battle droves of blackflies in spring, plant and weed our quarter-acre vegetable garden annually, and of course regularly chop kindling for the woodstove fires, our primary source of heat. The well can run dry for stretches on end in a summer drought, and winter storms often knock out power for days, leaving us to rely on candles, the woodstove, and resourcefulness.

Our lives are imbued with a richness of spirit and heart, in spite of the extra physical work. It feels right to raise our children amid fairy houses made of feathered hemlock boughs and to leave our summertime back door perpetually open, as sunshine and fresh air seep into our bed pillows and hearth. Sometime in June we toss aside our shoes, padding barefooted and carefree throughout the remaining unencumbered, golden days. I tuck a pair of moccasins under my driver's seat in the car, kept on hand for a dash into the market. Otherwise, we traipse on calloused soles down to the lakefront for a swim or into a friend's yard, natural and free-spirited.

Life here in this comely township is turning out to be pretty cozy. Though the big cities and their cultural enrichment are ninety minutes or more away, I have come to enjoy country living. Gourmet restaurants and brand-name shopping we do not have. The major department stores are a good distance away. I do miss my ethnic clan and all the love that flows so openly, but we trade traffic snarl and cloying smog for immense natural beauty and a well-fostered simplicity.

Until now I have not regretted my move to the north woods, despite my family's dismay. But I'm beginning to have concerns. Something doesn't feel right inside me again. My arms are aching at painting class. In fact, I'm tired and fuzzy-headed most all the time. I find myself sitting in a chair trying to paint, which I have never done before, because standing three hours becomes exhausting. Then I miss a few classes. Shockingly, I don't sign up for the winter painting session. Instead, I spend my time riddled with worry about the upkeep of our physical lifestyle with my energy flagging. The children are still too young to manage chores. Plus I am losing a strong ally.

We bid Sophie farewell in the harried days approaching Christmas. Her year with us has flown by and we have all grown to love her. She became a big sister to the children, gleefully running alongside Eli as he learned to master his two-wheeler, whooping when he successfully traversed the yard. The endless hours on the swing set, braiding Sarah's long hair, and all the help laundering and with chores. Sophie has been a huge helpmate to me, keeping our home life, our routines, and the structure of our days intact. Plus she witnessed me get well and learn to paint. My fondness for her and my gratitude are everlasting. Now, our dear Sophie flies off to New York City to work for another family and eagerly meet up with her new Czech boyfriend, found on the Internet. How will I manage without her? We send Sophie off with hugs and teary good-byes in the snow-filled driveway, an armload of Christmas gifts adorning her.

"Ciao, ciao." We wave in farewell as the car descends the hill, Sophie crying in the backseat.

Meanwhile, the weakness returns, the migraines intrude, the insomnia stomps its ugly feet, and my stomach lurches in burning pains. Eli has started preschool. The road appears wavy to me as I weave my way the five miles to pick him up at noontime. Once again I close up shop in my office. *How can all this be coming back?* I fret. I thought I had beaten this virus. It's been seven months of good health.

But down, down, down I fall, sinking into the quicksand of illness, disappointment, and confusion. The crying returns, so does the frustration. I find myself curled up and sobbing in the wee hours of the night or bursting out in irritability over a broken can opener at lunchtime. I'm trying to paint as in days past, upstairs in the biscuit-colored light of my studio. Nothing is going well, though. My head spins, the paintbrush is sloppy in my hands, and the colors look murky.

As we ring in 2002, I am forlorn.

The Meeting

January is the bleakest month of the year. Truncated days of blanched sunlight and sub-zero temperatures span for weeks in a row, as snows pound the region in habitual fashion. We bundle the children in down-and-fleece wrappings before turning them loose into winter's playground.

Today Eli and his sled have gone wayward in one blazing run over a man-made jump crafted by the big kids. While a dozen happy children zoom and traipse up and down this especially fine sledding hill, my independent four-year-old is brambled in a thicket of bushes. I try to finesse him out of the deep snow crater.

"No, Mommy!" he insists. "I can do it."

I extend my arm as far as I can reach down into the three-foot-deep crevasse, trying to tug him upward.

"Eli, you are way down in there. I can't really reach you, honey. Let me come in and push you up from behind."

My head pounds in wicked shards of pain. It's another migraine. How fierce they are again. This is the third one this week, plundering my body and mind, making it difficult to think or to speak, let alone to tend to my family. I wish that Joel were home to take over for me, to be out here on the sledding hill in fifteen-degree weather. But he is away on a work trip, not due back till close to midnight. Meanwhile,

I'm living on handfuls of ibuprofen, which merely dull the edge of the excruciating pain.

Up comes Eli over the crater's edge, his determined mouth suddenly smiling in triumph.

"Wow, Eli! You were right," I congratulate him. "You could get out of there on your own."

I know how physically focused this mighty pint of a boy can be. He runs and tugs his sled from the bushes and starts the ascent back up the looming hill. With each step behind him in the thigh-high snow, my head pounds in deliriums of pain, limbs aching in fatigue.

When I awaken the next morning, the migraine persists. I've been ransacked by these especially vile attacks since November. It feels like meningitis, the pain sears so brutally. The entire left side of my head and neck are inflamed with icepick-stabbing pain. Light, sound, a slamming cupboard door all exacerbate the blistering pain to the point of hysterical tears. Ice packs swaddling my head, I lie propped on pillows in bed, the shades drawn, my life falling away again, and me feeling very sorry for myself. I came to accept the monthly hormonal migraine headaches a decade ago, but this recent hurricane is just too overpowering to bear. I am worn to the bone.

"Joel, do you think I could have a brain tumor?" I weep.

"Probably not," he tries to reassure me, "but get yourself to the doctor. I hate seeing you suffer like this. There must be a reason for this outbreak."

He's right. Information always helps. I have struggled with migraines for a long time, though not as fierce as these, and the most interesting help I've come across wasn't from a doctor at all.

Way back in 1988, still married to Ray and living on the glamorous North Shore of Long Island, I stumbled one day upon a small miracle of a book in a local shop. It was a modern-day Carlos Castaneda–type story about a remarkable woman's personal experience of spiritual awakening. At the time I was shaken up by the fact that a so-called normal woman—a housewife and mother, living just across Long Island Sound—had her life turned inside out when a being in spirit form entered her life during her meditations, bringing messages and guidance. I was simultaneously fascinated and scared that something so unusual and profound could occur to anyone other than a priest, monk, or mystic. Despite my fear, I told friends about this fascinating book and inwardly longed to meet this clearly notable woman, who inspired me with her obvious gifts of wisdom.

The years passed as I made my new life in New Hampshire. All the while, I was plagued by monthly migraines. I tried all sorts of natural health-care approaches, chiropractic, herbs, reflexology, cranial sacral therapy, on and on, with only minor success. I found that homeopathy brought me the best relief, though even that was only temporary. Eventually, in desperation, I resorted to pharmaceuticals to squelch the savage pain. My friends knew how I suffered.

One day, a colleague of mine, Elizabeth, invited me to go to a Sunday meditation circle with her in a neighboring township. "It's led by an amazing woman," she said. "Meredith is an intuitive healer, a medical clairvoyant. In fact, she does readings about your health if you want help with the migraines. You'll like her, Kim."

"Meredith who?" I asked.

"Meredith Young-Sowers. She wrote *Agartha: Journey to the Stars*. Did you ever read it?"

My jaw dropped. I was momentarily frozen.

"What? She lives near us?" I practically screeched. "I thought she lived in Connecticut."

"No, she lives in Palmer. She has for some time now. She and her second husband have a lovely place on the hillside, with the most glorious gardens. It's gorgeous. You'll love it there. Come with me this Sunday."

I was stunned to learn that this woman I had been so taken by ten years prior, whom I had longed to one day meet, was a mere thirty minutes from me now. Unfortunately, my prior plans prevented me from joining Elizabeth for the Sunday meditation circle, but I called and made an appointment to see Meredith on my own for an intuitive healing session.

A few weeks later, on a sunny, fragrant spring day, with blooming apple trees dotting the roadside, I drove to Stillpoint, Meredith's center. Meeting Meredith felt natural and comfortable. Her warmth, love, compassion, and clarity wafted over me with grace and beauty. We sat together in her breezy garden, birds singing in full fanfare. Her aqua-blue eyes glowed as sharp as gemstones.

Meredith spoke to me about the migraines and her intuitive understanding of why my body was running this haywire pattern. She felt that it was all tied into my endocrine system, my pituitary gland specifically, and a certain piece of trauma about being unglued from my birth family and now living so far removed from my roots up here in New Hampshire. She spoke to me at length, too, about the recent loss of my mother and how that related to my hormonal chemistry. She offered some therapeutic ideas and gave me two healing exercises to implement at home, to help steady the hormonal fluxes and assuage the grief over my mom.

As Meredith walked me out to my car, she said, "Kim, I've started a school to train intuitive healers. I'd like you to consider joining us in the program at Stillpoint. I can see how strong your natural intuition is. You're a fine candidate to learn this work, especially with all your experience in homeopathy. I think you'd like it."

I was honored and flabbergasted all at once. "Really?" I asked.

"Oh, yes," she said, "you'd fit in beautifully."

Unfortunately, with a one-year-old only just weaned and a husband who traveled extensively, I realized that the timing was wrong to pursue such a program. I also had a large homeopathic practice to focus on. With constant demands placed on me at all times, taking time out for schooling would have been an unaffordable luxury. Sadly, I had to defer.

"But what a wonderful notion it is!" I said in parting to Meredith. "Maybe in a couple of years it could work out."

"Yes, dear heart. When the time is right, you'll know. I'll be here, don't worry," she said, smiling in her knowing, luminous way. "I'll see you again."

I floated home, the car coasting over back roads, the verdant hills shimmering in sprays of sunshine. I felt blessed in some way, as if I had been in the presence of an angel. Meredith's energy was so nurturing, kindly, and understanding. How I ached to go to her school. Like so much else, this wish had to be shelved while I worked on the immediate needs of my current place in life. Like a good worker bee, I had to keep our household and careers in motion. The wish fell to the wayside.

Now, prostrate in my bed and drugged up on pharmaceuticals that bring no real relief, I muse once again on Meredith's opinion about my pituitary gland and my being unglued from my roots. Ill yet again and racked in ferocious pain, I feel even more isolated and detached from my New York family. I wonder whether my chemistry has gone haywire. Worried, profoundly weak, and too sick to function in a daily capacity, I cart myself back to the doctor for testing.

Nora orders a brain MRI scan and other lab tests. Within short order I learn that I do not have a brain or pituitary tumor, but, as before, the Epstein-Barr titres are very high.

"It's reactivated infection," Nora says. "You're back in an active phase of the virus, Kim. Bedrest and minimal stress for six weeks. I want you to see a neurologist at Dartmouth to get some relief with this migraine pattern. You may need a new medication. I will call and set an appointment for you."

"I just said good-bye to the au pair two weeks ago!" I cry, exasperated. "How am I going to manage this whole mess again? Eli is only four years old. I've been sick forever!"

I feel profoundly frightened and just plain defeated. How can this be happening...and why?

The Doldrums

Our property line is marked by snow-dirndled conifers, which stand in convivial clusters marking the borders of my world. I admire their union as I struggle in a lonesome longing of my own. Lumbering through the heaving days of winter, my spirits fall very low, my body empty and pained. Since the rapid downhill slide of my vitality a few months ago, each week drives me deeper into the morass of illness. The neurologist has found a newer drug to squelch the migraine attacks to a degree, but the hazy, cotton-filled feeling in my head builds thicker and thicker, leaving me dazed and vaporous, struggling to find a simple name or noun I really do know. My once lightning-bright mind grapples with a grocery list. It's frightening, really. Forty-three is too young for this sort of slippage.

Somehow, I stumble along, minding my four-year-old as he bounces happily on the cushioned floral sofa, singing "The Wonderful Thing about Tiggers" again and again. My limbs are limp, deadened, and log-like as I lie on the floor, helping Eli fit the wooden train tracks together in his vastly elaborate designs. Our entire downstairs living space is covered with twisting, arching extensions of his Thomas the Tank Engine train set. With his budding mind, vast in vision and ambition, Eli builds while I collapse.

Who knows where the days and nights go? I'm in a fog, a dreary fog, pressing me down into the deepest, most forlorn well of my life. I see no one other than my immediate family. Joel and Sarah flit in and out to work and school, friends and errands. I feel stranded, literally and figuratively, deep in the woods, deep in the illness, deep in my loneliness. By now my friends have dwindled to close to nil. Charlene, bless her heart, still gathers groceries on occasion. But the mothers in my weekly playgroup are busy with lives of their own, their preschoolers and older children occupying so many of their hours. And in reality, though I wouldn't admit it to the au pairs, we live in the woods, outside of town, not quite as easy to reach us as I had perceived. The isolation is now bearing down on me, too.

Coupled with this drowning misery is an intense and unexplained anxiety. For no specific reason or obvious trigger, a growing frantic feeling will start inside. The vibrations initially roil in my lower back, making me feel jumpy and edgy. After an hour or so, they climb, like a vine up a garden trellis, wrapping around my spine, through my stomach, and locking into my chest. There the disagreeable energy sits, jittering and then thunderous. Finally, panic and fear gnaw into my head. Thoughts race. It can arise anytime, any situation, no rhyme or reason: lying in a warm tub, watching a PBS children's show, awakening me from sleep. I feel vulnerable, fragile, confused, and alarmed.

What is going on inside me? This is nuts! Me, the stalwart sailor who could jibe my Sonar sailboat, crisp as a knife's edge, in the dead heat of a wind-fraught race, now can barely manage preparing a meal. It's maddening to feel my mind and body so out of my control. But there is a pattern. These spells run a six-week cycle and then flag into an even deeper exhaustion and depression. I see a sequence to it all, feel the chemical yo-yo.

And, all the while, I keep telling my doctor, my neurologist, my gastroenterologist that I feel something in my blood. It sits in my neck and shoulders. It feels sicky, like a bug, a germ, or a bacterium. I can feel it. My neck is killing me, all stiff and swollen, the migraines playing tag team. I visit the chiropractor constantly. The anxiety grows when I get that germy, sicky feeling.

My descriptions are met with nods and dim looks.

"I swear there's something in my bloodstream," I tell them. I know how healthy I was before all this. I was the picture of vitality and ambition, glowing with energy. While all the clients in my office were hacking on me with bronchitis and strep, I would never get a thing. My immune system was so strong. I caught a little cold maybe once per year. Now I can feel this bug in me!

The doctors shrug it off. My finely tuned instincts aren't valued or explored. Instead, I'm told that I'm run down, that I have chronic fatigue syndrome, and that I need to rest, which I have been doing for close to two steady years now. I'm given Xanax, valerian, and other tranquilizers to settle my fraying nervous system. I take one at bedtime and at least find some steady sleep, by now a much-needed commodity.

But I still struggle so acutely. My life feels destroyed in so many ways. I've closed up shop on my illustrious homeopathic office, having passed on my clientele to two homeopaths in neighboring states. I can no longer ski or hike, run or canoe. Long gone are the dinner parties, snowball fights with the children, Latin dancing with my husband. Ugly words and angry voices now hurl through the house. Joel and I are tethered to one another in a fun-house mirror of emotional distortion. I no longer know what is up or down. My bearings are completely askew. Friends and rotating babysitters help to bolster our broken home life, doing the laundry and shopping for us, playing with the kids, trying to pick up some of the pieces of our shattered world. It's all so overwhelming.

Joel grows angry and distant. His once dynamic, capable, and rather charming wife lies flat and hollow month after month, horizontal on the sofa, bed, or floor. He's frustrated at my inability to be the wife he needs me to be. Joel spews out at Eli in volcanic eruptions, not being able to handle the whimsy, the burgeoning independence, the spurts of resistance in a growing four-year-old. I cringe, I cry, I wrap my arms around my little boy. He, too, fears Mommy's evaporation. We all do, really. Where am I going to? What is making me disappear in so many ways? Silently, we all are afraid. How can a healthy, holistically oriented woman change so radically for no diagnosable reason other than Epstein-Barr outbreaks? Intuitively, this all feels wrong to me. I took such great care of myself, balanced my life with conscious choice, eating organic food from my garden, meditating, exercising regularly, using natural medicine, and avoiding chemical drugs. This all seems so much bigger than being run-down and succumbing to EBV outbreaks, I think to myself.

In order to make it through, I visit either the acupuncturist's or kinesiologist's office each week. They are the only ones able to give me a slight energy lift for a day or two. Plus they supply me with a dose of encouragement.

"Your liver energy is just totally stagnant, Kim," my acupuncturist tells me again and again, "and your spleen energy is like a wet, soggy sponge." She says that my blood is shattered and insufficient, and that we need to generate more renewal there. I am instructed to cook thick bone soups and stews.

The pots begin to boil. I down endless teaspoons of bitter herbs, tonics, and teas. My vitamin arsenal at this time is mounting. Olive leaf extract is a huge staple for me, as it's known to kill off Epstein-Barr virus. I rely on a thymus glandular extract, too, to pump up my exhausted immune system. Adrenal support with vitamin C, licorice root, ginseng, and the almighty wonder of DHEA finally help me move from collapse to cooking again.

The loneliness mounts in proportion to the snows of the dark winter. As our post-and-beam home is blanketed deeper each week in the enveloping whiteness, I dive further into lassitude. The snow piles higher than the henhouse, up to my north-facing windowsills, burying even the tips of the tall garden fencing. All signs of former life and summer glory have vanished, just like me. The dead of winter. The dead of my life.

I look to my husband for emotional support. It's in very scant supply. Joel manages the running around, cooking, and carpooling with aplomb, his work schedule being self-regulated. He's able to handle desk and computer work at odd hours when we're all asleep. His travel is irregular, but known in advance. But I'm just so worn, on the edge of breaking. I crave caresses, hugs, steady words of encouragement, and confidence building. For Joel, this is the most impossible piece to muster, something truly not in his playbook of life and relationship skills. After all, he trains managers for a living; he does not do counseling work.

"Honey, can you spend just fifteen minutes a day with me? I feel so isolated and alone. I need some companionship," I ask.

"I have to do that?" comes the terse reply. He sounds legitimately flabbergasted.

My silent nod of affirmation feels pitiful and forlorn. How have I become so needy? Dependency does not become me. Why is this virus gripping me again and again? It's going on forever. Joel is trying hard to help me and the family, but this impasse of prolonged illness is breaking more than just me. He, too, is rattled. Heartbroken.

I'm beginning to recognize that I'm now heartbroken, too. The emptiness eclipses the fear. Sighs, shallow breaths, and a wobbly heartbeat set in. My spirit has been crushed. What is there to hold on to? No more than a filament of hope that I can live long enough to see the children safely grown and capable of surviving in the world.

I have been praying daily for months now, asking for guidance, support, and courage to make it through all this spiritually. I beseech the angels, my deceased mother's spirit, Mother Mary, and God to deliver me from this wicked ordeal. Little comes in direct response to my prayers. I feel abandoned by these honored masters of deliverance, too.

One miserable night in February, the sleet tapping on the skylight, I cry myself into a headache as Joel skims past me back into his sleep. Once again I fight the anxiety and the claw of tension in my chest. I pray from the deepest place in my heart, way down in the guts of my soul.

Please, God, I need to be loved with tenderness and compassion. My heart is broken. I need so much to have some TLC. It's what will cure me, I know this. Please bring it to me. Please! I need to see these children are raised with my love.

I feel I'm breaking in some inner way. I haven't much to hold on to now. I know I'm slipping down a cliffside I have not wanted even to face. I have held on to my emotions for twenty-one months. Now I'm cracking in a way I have forever dreaded. I hit bottom.

In late March, after a long, drawn-out winter of disharmonies, Joel, Eli, and I go see our family in Florida for a week. We hope that the sunshine will help me. Sure enough, the sun and salt work their magic and we head back north, my energy and spirits perking up. With April's arrival, we mark Eli's fifth birthday. Things seem to be looking up.

I make a wobbly trek down to Massachusetts to my homeopathic colleague and friend, Melinda. She has set up an appointment for me with a world-renowned master homeopath visiting from India. In years past I had studied with Jayesh; now I arrive as one of his patients. He spends a solid ninety minutes with me, exploring my case and reviewing my life history and these disconcerting years of poor health.

"You will be well again, Kim," he announces in his singsong voice. "Your constitution is prone to cyclical episodes of overactivity of the immune system, wearing you down to collapse. The homeopathic remedy will break that pattern and boost your resistance."

But, he tells me, I need to take caution and maintain a routine with maximum rest. He says that my finely tuned nervous system and brain need great peace and beauty.

"You must stop pushing yourself so hard," Jayesh instructs. "Someone besides you needs to manage money and trifles. Yours is a soul of compassion and creativity. You must nurture these strengths of yours. It will help you to be healthy and happy. Is your husband a strong businessman?"

I assure him that Joel is certainly that.

"Good. Let him focus on the outer world. You are blessed with a fine sensitivity, a true healer. A soul like you will shine brightly if you are physically secure so your inner riches are allowed to grow."

I nod, feeling deeply seen and validated by this man of eminent skill and keen observation.

Melinda and I feel greatly encouraged by Jayesh's remedy choice and his hopeful outlook. I pop the tiny white pellets under my tongue and creep up the roadway back to my home, with true faith that my cherished homeopathic medicine will work its wonders.

A week later I notice the magic beginning. My head starts to clear, my moods improve, and, slowly, with baby steps, I'm moving off the sofa. Once again, I feel optimistic that I'm rounding the corner, beating back the relentless virus. Up and down the hurdles of collapse and rebuilding I go. Physically renewed, I pick up my brushes and begin to paint with a refound passion. But despite all this, I know that a massive hemorrhage has erupted in my marriage.

Mastering the Mountain

Joel and I tumble in the chaos of our marital disharmony, fighting relentlessly over daily trifles, money, religion, parenting, responsibilities, and control. Sometimes, in the stilted hours of predawn, I lie empty in the haze of my confusion, imagining whether I could survive on my own, away from my known structure and security.

I wonder whether Eli and I could return to New York and my dad, or if we might stay in my girlfriend's guesthouse in Connecticut, where I could start up a new homeopathic practice. I try these notions on as escape-hatch alternatives to living in a stifling situation. All of it feels surreal and impossibly daunting to me, with my tender fragility and quaking low self-esteem. I talk to my counselor and close girlfriends, hoping to find a practical pathway out of my disenchantment. Nothing resonates as right, though. Jayesh told me that I need Joel's protection. Besides, I have a young son at my side and a pubescent stepdaughter woven into my heartstrings. How can I shatter their home life? So I stay on, holding steady under the titanic strains.

Consciously, with clear intention, I work daily to build up my physical strength and stamina, determined to regain my wholeness, even though trapped in the bungee cords of a now difficult marriage. I want desperately to feel well. With so many years in health care, I know how important it is to recondition my body and cardiovascular system. Since the slight upswing of energy after our Florida sojourn, I want to re-inforce this trend. So I pick a mountain to climb, a local one that has a lovely winding trail, a stunning westward view on the summit, and some fascinations of delicate wildflowers and Indian pipe en route. If I can master this mountain, perhaps I can master my illness and even my marriage.

And so it begins, my journey to the peak—to a place of beauty, a place of purpose, a place of completion. This I aim for with the ken of a seasoned archer. In the gentle mornings of May 2002, I don my well-worn, brown Vasque hiking boots, grab my felt fedora, call Echo into the car, and head off to the well-tramped trail of Bald Top Mountain. The first few attempts get us only a couple of football fields away from the car before my rasping breath and jangling limbs signal it's time to head back. But it's a start.

The carpet of mayflowers crowning the forest floor is green and wel-coming. My senses are fed by the dimples of sunshine dancing like spar-klers amidst the sheltering heavens of leaves overhead. Though I'm weak in body, my spirit is nurtured in this abundant wilderness. Sometime in the middle of July, Echo and I discover we are midway up a swiftly in-clining stretch of trail. It's a marvel to me how my strength is mounting. I see the frolicking stream bubble by, cascading downward over mossy logs and rounded rocks. I stop and sip the icy cold water. It's a milestone. I'm midway up the mountain, panting, sweaty, and, yes, doing okay! The marriage still ricochets, but my heart is working fine out here, deep in the woods.

All summer my faithful border collie and I address this feat of pur-pose. Two, three, even four times per week we inch further along this path of progress. I'm determined to put this illness and its devastations into their place. Frustration, willfulness, personal purpose, and eventu-ally enthusiasm fuel me onward. Step-by-step, day by day, I meet the earth, the sky, the summer air, welcoming them liberally into the swell-ing pockets of my tentatively healing spirit. As I slowly gain some physi-cal strength, my emotional body grows proportionately in volume.

Finally, it comes. Echo and I round a bend in the trail, amidst the stunted pines and low-growing blueberry bushes. I follow the rut-ted footpath as it transitions completely to aged granite, fissured with glacial cracks and speckled with glints of mica and blackened bits of weather. My senses lift a notch. I feel the cooling breeze of altitude, hear the white-throated sparrow's trill in the pine boughs, and welcome the sun's glare on my bare arms. Joyfully and with wild abandon, I'm scampering, yes, scampering, Echo running even faster and a few strides ahead of me, reaching the journey's end. We are there! I stand bold and emblazoned, in profound pride on the summit of my mountain peak. The world shimmers in a green glory far below me. Deliriously happy, I twirl around like an eight-year-old, sucking up the magnitude of my achievement. I bend and hug my dear Echo, knowing her treasured companionship has bolstered me along. I have mastered the mountain!

We sit a bit on the peak, soaking in our feat and the soothing horizon of violet-tinged, distant mountains. I spy the Presidential Range way up north and my favorite climb of them all, Mount Moosilauke, to the northwest. Some Triscuits, some water, an apple, and a handful of low- bush blueberries from beside me fill my stomach. The air is so sweet and pure. Echo lies quietly at my feet. I treasure the loveliness of it all. Eventually, it's time to head back to the car.

On the descent, back to the reality of my daily life, I'm buoyed in the euphoria and neurochemical rush of my personal achievement. It feels good, so satisfyingly good, to have worked four months and mastered the mountain. I can't help but reflect on the symbolism that I have elected to climb a mountain, not ride a bike, or swim a pond, but to tackle a task of great exertion and endurance both to improve my quality of health and to illustrate to myself that I can conquer a defeat. I'm musing on this concept as I come across an elderly, white-haired gnome of a man, gnarled walking stick in hand and head bent downward, studying the ground as he climbs.

"Hi there!" I say cheerfully.

Misty eyes peer up at me from behind wire-framed glasses. His shrunken shoulders are hunched forward.

"Good day, dear," he replies.

"Nice day for a hike."

"Certainly so. But I climb in all weather," he says.

"You do? Do you hike here often?"

"Regularly, you might say. Summer, winter, fall, and spring I'm out on the trails. I've been battling back leukemia."

My mind flip-flops. The only other hiker I come upon today happens to be another determined survivor on a quest like me.

"...been at it over six years now," he continues. "I won't let those wayward blood cells take me over. I find that exercise, particularly climbing in the outdoors, has fed me while the chemotherapy ransacks me."

"You are a true warrior," I say.

A small smile curls his lips. I tell him that today was a really big day for me, too.

We end up sharing the stories of our personal journeys through illness and back toward wellness, the kingdom of nature being our guide. We talk for a good fifteen minutes. This meeting on the trail feels more than coincidental to me. In fact, it strikes me as quite remarkable. We part with a hug and a sort of inner blessing toward one another. The true connection of spirit is threaded between us, woven with fellowship and understanding, a form of communion.

"You've done a great thing for yourself," he says. "Don't ever give up your dreams."

I smile in agreement.

"The view is lovely on top," I tell him in parting.

"It always is, my dear. Better than down at the bottom. Elevation has its way of broadening the picture for us. Remember, perspective can change everything."

I nod, absorbing his chestnut of advice.

"Have a good journey!" I call and start down the path. As I approach a scramble of rocks and tree roots, I look back to see the ancient one leaning on his staff, stepping with patience, steady and slow, up the steep trail.

In the upcoming weeks, as Indian summer days flourish in a fiesta of color and seventy-degree softness, I'm painting landscapes in a near frenzy. My energy is so much better than a year ago. The canvases fly from my fingertips, cloaked in scenes of the region. I'm soaring now in the outpouring of my creative endeavors and in the joy of realization that I have beaten back the illness. Tackling the mountain was a huge feat, but curing this illness is even bigger. My spirit rises with hope for my future.

Perspective can change everything, I think.

A Good-Bye

Eli ventures into kindergarten and, after a stellar seven weeks at sleepaway camp, a summertime of great joy and expansion, Sarah enters middle school. These are big steps for both our children. Unfortunately, Joel's work has dwindled and our income is scant. I've been able to maintain my bimonthly health column, with Joel helping with the typing, since the computer screen frazzles my mind. Still, we resort to a second mortgage on the house.

I decide to try seeing a few homeopathic clients once again, in hopes of rebuilding my practice and securing an income. Sadly, I struggle with managing others' health care. An extensive amount of mental application is required to determine which one of over four thousand homeopathic remedies is called for in each individual case, and my head buzzes like a beehive of confusion. The entire process drains me significantly. After a few weeks of effort, I must return home to quasi-invalid status. Stretched out on the sofa again, I fight the urge to just stay down forever.

A week or so into this plummet, I order myself to pick up my brushes. I bundle up in the hoarfrost-brittle mornings and ply the creamy paints into shadows and highlights on canvas, surveying the simplicity of our rural beauty. It does lift my spirits.

In the peak of the back-to-school flurry, our dear and sensitive Echo becomes unexpectedly ill. I come home from a windy painting outing to find large clumps of ebony fur falling off Echo into my hands. Over the next week, she is quiet and still, losing weight rapidly. Echo has never visited the vet in her eight years for any reason other than her annual checkup. She comes from sturdy, hardworking farm stock. All her relatives live into their mid-teens and are actually herding until the day they die. Ever loyal, her intelligent and emotive eyes hold mine in deep trust.

We find Echo has kidney failure. We are devastated. We try hand feeding her bits of bacon and salami, once her forbidden favorites. She won't eat anything. For the next two weeks I keep Echo with me constantly, lifting her in and out of the car, moving her from flower bed to flower bed with me as I plant fire-red tulips in the yard. I know these flowers will bloom next spring, reminding me of these final days with our family dog. Two days before her death I drive Echo to our mountain. Leaving her on blankets in the car, I kiss the white blaze on her forehead and tell her, "I'm climbing our mountain today just for you."

Tearfully, I sit on the familiar mossy patch at the summit, gazing out into the eternal blue without my faithful companion. It's the first time I have hiked alone without Echo. My heart aches with an unbearable heaviness. I feel the grief filling my chest in bucketfuls of disbelief.

Echo's last hours come on Halloween eve. She can no longer stand, whittled to mere skin and bones. What is left of her merely trembles. She has been resting in Eli's bedroom for days now. Joel, Sarah, Eli, and I sit in a circle around Echo cross-legged on the floor. We each individually take turns telling this dear one how we have loved her, what she has given us. It's touching and heartfelt. Sarah and I are sobbing as we prepare to take her to the vet for her final slumber.

On our front porch I give my beloved guardian her last kiss goodbye as she lies flaccid in Joel's strapping arms, under the glow of a chilly, star-filled night sky. Looking into the richness of Echo's ever-caring, tender eyes, I feel a ripping at my heart as she leaves my side for the very last time. All those hours she lay at my feet through illness, while nursing baby Eli, during bedtime books, the hikes, the skis, the eternal tending of the sheep and chickens, nipping at the UPS driver or warding off coyotes and foxes, Echo was ever faithful, ever proud. I sense the enormous emptiness we will feel with our girl gone, a hole in our family fabric without her.

The snows have come early this autumn. In the full peak of crimson-and-golden glory, large sopping white flakes cling to the jeweled trees. It sets one's orientation off kilter suddenly to find two seasons melded as one. By the time of Echo's passing, our ground is hardening quickly. On a stark, gray, early November afternoon we bury the body of our border collie alongside the large, flat, granite boulder right near the children's swing set.

I bend and snip off some of Echo's silky black-and-white fur for memories' sake and her stiffened body is foreign to my touch, her once playful energy stilled forever. We sing the lovely Shaker tune "Simple Gifts" and take turns shoveling the dark earth and ocher leaves over her. Our hearts hang low, orbs of emotion, delicate and glass-like, rimming our family's sorrow.

That night at bedtime I choke on a vitamin. No breath will go in or go out of my throat. No sound, no air. The vitamin is wedged, closing off my air pipes. In a sheer incline of fright, I'm pounding on the wall. Joel storms down the stairs, and Heimlichs me two times without success. My mind is racing in a near-death hallucination.

Am I dying, too? Panic surges through my veins. Joel slaps my back with full force. I lurch forward from the impact. The pill pops out onto the floor. In a choking, gasping stretch for air I collapse into Joel's arms.

"I'm still good for something," he jokes.

Death, however, is knocking at our door. It's frightening, actually. A tangible energetic presence has insidiously slipped its way into our lives. Something in my awareness tells me that the energy of death rode its ugly face in on those cold north winds of October, as that sudden unpredicted snowstorm trounced us. Like a cloying fog, death hangs in the air of our rooms. I can taste it, feel it on my skin, moist and clinging. I light candles and burn sage in front of the small photo of Echo now on an altar, hoping to drive out this unnerving presence.

In the pinched light of descending winter, we round the bend toward Christmastime. I sense the suggestion of weakness and fatigue in my bones and load up on my vitamins and homeopathic remedies. Staving off the virus feels critical to me now.

Twist of Fate

One frosted winter's eve I wander into a party and run into a former client of mine from years past. Hunter Baldwin had come to me eight years prior with his one-year-old daughter swaddled in his arms. This saucer-eyed, cute-as-punch baby was afflicted with brain cancer. Against beseeching pleas from my empathic secretary, I had adamantly refused to take on any cancer cases, even one as heart-wrenching as this one. I relented, finally agreeing to work only on strengthening this youngster's immune system with homeopathy, not treating the cancer at all.

For three years I helped Blue through her chemo and radiation treatments. She fared remarkably well: Blue kept her hair, never lost weight, and maintained rosy cheeks when the other children battling cancer around her suffered miserably. In fact, she had miraculously defied the odds of the six-month death sentence she'd been given at the outset.

Her father stood out in my mind, too, as rather impressive. In my many years of practice I had never encountered a man who had taken on the role of primary caretaker of an ill child. Hunter was smart, attentive, very nurturing, and obviously devoted to his daughter. Together, we worked through many of Blue's woes, from radiation burns, nausea, and rashes, to obsessive nail biting and more, with homeopathy's gentle ministerings assuaging many of her discomforts.

By the time they left my orbit when Blue was around age four, I was delighted to watch a smiling, cancer-free, auburn-haired cherub walk outside onto the sun-splashed grass all on her own. I recall the awareness I had then, that this was one of those handfuls of cases that would stay within me forever. I felt a deep fulfillment in my heart, knowing I had helped someone so intrinsically. I saw homeopathy do its best with this little girl and I felt proud of my skills.

Naturally, the first question out of my mouth these years later is, "How is Blue?"

"Oh, she's great," he beams. "She's eleven now, in fifth grade, and healthy."

My heart soars for them. Hunter and I continue to talk for a bit. After eight years it's nice to catch up on their lives. He suggests it might be nice for me to see Blue again, all these years later, as a buoyant and healthy schoolgirl.

"I like that idea. How about we meet for lunch one day?" I suggest.

A few weeks later I am reintroduced to a shy but happy young girl with the same brown eyes and steady demeanor. We chat over tuna sandwiches, me learning about her dog and friends, favorite colors and TV shows. What an inspiration she is, I think.

A few weeks later, however, I receive a phone call from Hunter. His voice is clearly tense.

"Kim, I have bad news. At Blue's annual MRI they found tumor activity; apparently, the cancer has returned. Can you help her?"

Sadly, I tell him why I can't. "I'm not strong enough yet to take on clients again," I tell him. "But I can give you a referral to a terrific homeopath. She's one of the best in New England."

"But you've been through so much with us, Kim," he reasons. "No homeopath knows Blue as well as you do."

It breaks my heart, but I must be adamant—for Blue's sake, as well as my own. I assure Hunter that they will like Melinda. "She's great," I promise. "Smart, sensitive, keen minded, and talented. She's very caring, too, and only one hour away."

He reluctantly takes her phone number and I tell him that I'll forward Blue's file.

I feel awful for them, but the strange thing is I'm aware of a knowing instinct rising in my gut. This is why they have returned into my life, these two, out of the beyond. For some reason, I'm supposed to see this little girl through to the end. *Is it destiny?* A haunting feeling sits with me for the next several days.

Within the week Hunter calls again. "I know you can't see Blue, but at least can you help me get the old remedies straight?" he asks.

They have an appointment to see Melinda and he wants to meet with me in person to go over the details of our previous treatments.

I feel for them and figure thirty minutes of my time won't be too much. Hunter is extremely grateful. I can see it written all over his sad face on the day of our informal appointment. I wish him the best as he heads off in his white Taurus station wagon, the deep snowbanks spiring above his roofline in the ominous winterscape.

Over the next few weeks Hunter calls me regularly, initially with an update after seeing Melinda, eventually with a question or merely a note on Blue's status. Soon the phone conversations become more familiar and conversational, a chord of friendship building. Between the lines I sense a loneliness in him.

As the snows endlessly pound us in billowing spring storms, it becomes apparent that the brain tumor is not growing. "Blue is just as normal as usual," Hunter conveys to me. "She's showing no symptoms at all."

"Well, keep me informed," I say, and he says that he will.

The two of them vanish from my sphere once again.

Vernal Equinox

Though my health is holding, my marriage feels more fractured than ever. I spend months wracked by confusion and upset. Nothing seems right between Joel and me anymore. Fights flare without any warning. We bicker even in the therapist's office. Everything we once had in common is now in turmoil. We have no steady income. In the aftermath of the 9/11 attacks, Joel's work has dwindled to a standstill and mine is gone, the office closed up. The house is double mortgaged. I have gouged into my retirement savings. My health is so fragile that we can no longer ski or canoe together, nor entertain. Our social life is at a halt, which is tough on two extroverts. I am struggling with huge issues, scissored between conflict and fear. Joel and I both retreat deeper into isolation and resentment. My heart is bleeding in sorrow as I recall the incandescent glow of our snowcapped wedding. I mastered a mountain, but I cannot master this marriage.

I see now that terrific omen of the enormous bleeding heart in Joel's garden on the evening we met. There it looms, abundant and full, achingly beautiful on a still summer's night—a shimmering memory. I have been betrayed by my body, by the medical world, and now by love. This is when I taste a new kind of fear. I pray at bedtime and at dawn, for guidance and protection to help find my way, but my defeat feels as inescapable as the icy tooth of winter.

As spring finally pokes its tender breath into our lives, we are worn to ragged edges in many ways. Besides enduring a winter of Nordic proportions, our emotional dynamics are even more troubled. I realize I'm holding on to my marriage by mere fingertips. The thought of ripping order, security, and comfort from my two children's lives hurts me.

It has been quite a feat finessing timid Eli through kindergarten. He has struggled with leaving our homespun feathery nest since preschool. Sarah may be more resilient, yet it is awful to imagine how her world will be wrenched should Joel and I separate. I soldier on, though, my mind constantly whirling in broken pathways. The fact is that I'm scared, confused, and very, very tired.

Rebuilding my health becomes a stabilizing focal point. *A strong body builds a strong heart and mind,* I keep reminding myself. Prayer and meditation become my security blanket, along with my daily practice of yoga. Stretching, breathing, and leaning my body in various asanas on my cranberry-colored mat, I attempt to knit together some sort of vigor and strength within. I earnestly make my way to the pool, too. Lap after lap, the rhythmic breathing uncurls the crimped knots of my heartstrings. Breathe and blow, breathe and blow. The mantra drones in my mind as my arms circle round in freestyles and backstrokes of repetition. The minutes fly by, the aquamarine blue endures. If life could only be as free and easy as swimming laps, I think. I hurt, though. So much of me hurts: my heart, my body, and my mind.

The sun has reached its equilibrium point on the vernal equinox. The air is softening, the light expanding. I prepare my canvases for my first plein-air outing of the year and feel like a filly at the paddock gate, my senses heightened, my energy impetuous and erratic, ready to bolt outdoors into the vast tableau of nature. My hands are literally itching to paint, my spirit aching to express itself in color.

I run to the snow-dimpled, soggy fields, oblivious to the mud and blunt light, craving the song of yellow ochers and alizarin crimson as they blend together in bloody arrays on my stark wooden palette. The first few canvases are rather awkward, the colors too vibrant, the farmhouse a bit stiff. It doesn't really matter, however. It's a start for the season, and the sap is running both in the tall, gnarly sugar maples and in the veins of my body. Painting enlivens me. It's my alcohol in a way, lifting me beyond my worries and woes into a neurochemical surge of heightened senses.

Over the next few weeks, the greening days and robin-filled skies cajole me into planting a few rows of vegetable seeds, needing to feel a new beginning after endless months of woodsmoke and dry air. The old-timers in these parts tell us not to waste early efforts: "Don't plant until Memorial Day, after the threat of heavy frost has passed." But the stirrings within the earth call to me. Tilling the fresh soil on an April morning, the rhythmic raking and turning motions stretch my winter-crimped muscles, awakening now in the leafless light. By morning's end I have flung myself on the fragrant loam, sweat and fatigue melding with Mother Earth's moisture and dark-brown silkiness. Breathing in the earthen aroma, all the pent-up tensions of the trying months in darkness and cold slowly melt away. I shed tears of relief into the soil, sensing the blessedness of renewal.

Sure enough, the frosts arrive on a stolen spring night, scouring the seeds and trampling down the tendrils of sprouts. On another morning I'm in a state of semi-shock to find heavy, lavender lilacs draped downward like nuns at prayer, their glorious blooms coated with two inches of unexpected snow. But eventually, if I'm patient, the brimming vegetable garden will feed us through the summer and deep into the winter months.

And, one fine day, the brilliant red tulips I so lovingly planted last fall bloom in a delirium of color. I stand quietly beside them, tears brimming against my eyelashes as I remember how our beautiful Echo lay next to me as I planted them. My heart hangs heavy and low. I walk over to her grave site and sit beside her remains, on the table-sized boulder. The swing set is stationary, the children at school. Somewhere out of sight, the chickens are scratching. I hear their soft rustle in the dried leaves. Greenery sprouts in the woods and the yard. I study the delicate curlicues of the succulent fiddleheads at my ankles. The world revolves in its endless Ferris wheel of seasons and consistency. For all that appears good, I still feel broken.

The Ride

On a clear day late in spring, having battled droves of blackflies for too many hours, I call it quits at the easel and head home early. Turning up the hill into my driveway, I glimpse something Ferrari red and white coming down the road in the opposite direction. Soon I hear the grumbling growl of a motorcycle engine behind me. Stepping out of my Jeep, I find the machine in my driveway, the helmeted driver dismounting.

"Let's go for a ride," the cyclist calls to me, the engine now purring at an idle.

I'm caught off guard. Swooped up in the fanciful notion of a masked man appearing on such a steed at my doorstep and boldly inviting me to take off with him, I feel a spontaneous rush fly through me. I peer through the helmet visor, trying to see who this leather-clad road warrior might be. He obviously senses my confusion, because he flips up the visor, brown eyes flickering in merriment. Off comes the helmet, revealing the suddenly sexy smile of Mr. Hunter Baldwin, his dark hair ruffled and careless.

"Oh, hi. It's you!" I warble, trying to sound nonplussed.

"It's a beautiful day. Come for a spin," he says.

"Is this your bike?"

"No, it's a friend's. He sent me to town on it for an errand. I figured you'd like to take a ride. It's a gorgeous machine."

He's right; it's a gorgeous machine, big, powerful, glistening, bold, and beckoning me. "But will he mind you giving me a ride?"

"God, no! What's an extra ten minutes?"

"Do you have another helmet?" I ask, suddenly insecure. Yet the bike's purr is seducing me by the second.

"No, but you can wear this one." He hands me the bright-red and black sphere in his left hand. "I'll be fine without one just down the road and back."

By now my heart is racing. I love motorcycles. I always have. My first husband had two, and we rode most weekends. It has been almost a decade now since I've been on the back of a two-wheeled wonder like this.

"Okay," I announce, the risk taker in me sparking to the surging adrenaline rush. It's as if I'm coming alive after a long, gauzy sleep. The free-spirited tomboy in me has lain dormant these past two years, yet here I am straddling a seat behind a new friend, swooping off into the teeming day.

We zoom up the road, cresting the ridge, coasting down the long hill, then gliding swiftly through the hemlock and oak tree shadows. My arms are wrapped tightly around Hunter's strong torso, my chest pressed against his back. The bike vibrates in its throaty tremolo beneath me. The air whips my hair. Colors stream by. I'm momentarily frightened about crashing, but I talk myself out of it. We veer into a hard corner. I follow Hunter's body language, leaning into the turn, as my father taught me to do as a good backseat rider decades ago. I relax into the thrill of it all. It's exciting, fun, and a bit improper.

Who cares! I internally scream. *It's my life. I can do this if I want to.* But I do wonder just how pissed off my husband will be if he discovers me out on a motorcycle with another man.

Fortunately, we're back home again in a few minutes. I say a swift good-bye to Hunter, grab my wet paintbrushes from the car, and dash into the house, my heart still beating at a gallop. Ten minutes of head-spinning dare has thrown me sky high, like a twirling baton, out and above the ruts of my predictable life.

I have thirty minutes till Eli's school bus arrives, which gives me some time to settle down. I coerce myself into a modicum of steadiness. But what has been planted is a simple seed of potential within me. As I wash my boar bristle brushes at the sink, a trickle of forewarning meanders through my mind. Those ten renegade minutes have rattled open a firmly shuttered window in my heart.

Is it possible that I could have fun in my life again? There are thoughtful and caring men in the world. It doesn't have to be all business and lists, sickness and details, does it?

Suddenly, I feel like a schoolgirl, caught up in the daydream of escaping from my own life and riding off into the sunset into a new one. By the next morning I'm ashamed of myself for allowing my mind to run so wild. But, oh, what fun the joyride was!

Bird Nesting

In July of 2003 Joel and I actually do separate. The divorce battle begins, the lawyers are installed, the swords are drawn, and the first cuts ooze blood. I sense we will not die a quiet death. It will be long and drawn out—apocalyptic.

The dance draws on into the dark hours of seamless nights and strings of endless days. I continue to cry, trying hard to say good-bye to this great love of mine. After loving so deeply, it is wrenching to let go. I know that it will take me years to recover.

In the meantime I put my heart and soul into my six-year-old son. We both have so much to adjust to. Eli has always been insecure. Joel and I both realize that this divorce will shake his core. And poor Sarah, having to deal with another divorce, reshuffling her deck of cards in life once again. At thirteen she may cope better than she did at four. Still, it's a chasm I hate to see her cross. Blessedly, Sarah has the security of her mother's home and love to shore her up. Eli does not have that extra support.

I pray that the children will be cushioned from the inevitable blows. *Please, please, spare Eli and Sarah!* I call out silently. *I'll take the hit.*

The years ahead will be rocky for the kids. Joel and I both know that from here on it will be damage control. Our therapist has counseled us to employ a method called bird nesting in an effort to ease the kids into this transition.

Our children will stay in the family home during the first few months of the separation, and we adults will alternate living with them, each of us flitting in and out like bird parents, who take turns feeding and caring for their young. This is believed to provide a softer transition for children coping with the shock of losing their family structure. As the tidewaters of the divorce ebb and the reality sets in that Mom and Dad can no longer live together, each parent eventually stays put in their new dwelling, and the children start making the dual-home trek between them.

Joel and I devise a half-week bird-nest schedule, each staying with the children in our family home for three days, and then alternating. It's a bit chaotic, but okay in a way. We scribble notes to one another about laundry and the garden, camp schedules and chores. The grocery list dangles from the fridge door, littered with both Joel's and my handwriting. Our personal belongings are still intact, the furniture and art unmoved. These familiar items are unchanged in the children's eyes. It's just that Mom and Dad are rarely at home together anymore.

Joel and I cross paths on transition days. I summon up my bubbly persona, always projecting a happy image to the kids. I don't want them to see me sad or frayed. They saw too much of that when I was so ill. Now that they must cope with the divorce, I want them to feel as little worry, fear, and insecurity as possible.

I try to prompt within their conscience the idea that if Mommy looks and feels good, then they can feel good, too. Who knows if this is truly effective? I give it a try anyway, knowing that kids take their cues from adults. These times are wrenching, painful, and consuming. But part of me insists that I have to break away from Joel and the old life. Something unseen audaciously propels me forward.

Now, with the shackles of a troubled marriage lifting from me, I'm infused with a vibrancy and vitality reminiscent of the true me. I'm laughing again, freely. I'm lighter, sillier, more enthused about everything. During my three days at the house, I'm playing baseball in the yard with Eli and his friends, and hosting cookouts. When I'm away from the house, I'm dancing in the local pub and selling my paintings at shows. No more sickness. I have energy to hold me. What a boon!

Eli's been meeting some of my new friends. We invite people to dinner often and swim together at the pond. It seems I've become a social butterfly. Many men in town are paying attention to me. It's nice to suddenly find myself being invited to parties, out to dinner, or to the county fair. Hunter has become one of these new friends. I'm finding that life in the single fast lane at forty-five is more liberating than I would've imagined. The daring intrepidness of my launch into the New Hampshire woods twelve years ago has returned. I feel heedless, giddy, and youthful. This surge toward independence drives me far and wide. As Eli nears first grade, both his and my heart alight on the wings of discovery.

The New World

I continue to paint when I can, squeezing it into the tiny jug-
gernauts of space between health-care appointments, house chores, and
general life as a single mother. I've lost many friends in these months
of our marital separation. I'm more alone now psychically, but it's an
exciting and challenging time in my life. The keynote, however, is that
the Epstein-Barr virus seems to have gone dormant. It has been one
solid year of vastly improved energy, minimal gastrointestinal upset, less
frequent headaches, and, miraculously, no naps needed. The blood work
finally shows the virus is in remission.

Am I finally cured? I wonder. *Could it be that the endorphins and immune-
enhancing hormones of a blossoming love affair are buoying my health?*

Hunter and I have discovered that we share a wonderful synergy.
His laid-back Wyoming steadiness counterbalances my spitfire tendencies. I engage him, stimulate him, and propel him out of his comfort
zone. Meanwhile he grounds me, slows down my lightning-strike im-
petuousness, and quells my jittery nerves. We find a deep kindred bond
in our love of the outdoors. Whether we're hiking or stargazing, a sense
of perfect peace drifts into our hearts, forming a palpable, unspoken
bond. We're both affectionate and nurturing—and we both happen to
love the Boston Red Sox. Throw in his streak of "bad boy" daring and

my headstrong ambition, and our mixture brews a passionate chemistry. The fire between us ignites.

Hunter is staying, rent free, in a crazy, ramshackle house in exchange for his carpentry work. The curving bay window and Victorian porch are lovely, yet the place is very worn. I stay there with him sometimes during the half week of bird nesting when Joel is living at our house with the kids.

"My mother would have a heart attack if she saw me staying in this joint," I tell him.

Hunter says nothing, but holds my hand tightly.

The place is funky, to say the least. There's no electricity except for one lightbulb working in the downstairs bath. Hunter hauls in an old refrigerator, as there are no kitchen appliances. We cook on a camping stove until it blows up in a fiery ball one evening, sending me screaming out of the house in a panic, terrified that this tinderbox will burn down. The floors are sanded, yet unstained, and covered with stretches of brown paper. The only furniture is a queen-sized mattress and box spring, and a rummage-sale kitchen table with chairs.

The upstairs rooms are cordoned off, sequestering mountains of boxes crammed with antiques and old books. The house feels a bit spooky with its nineteenth-century windows rattling in the updraft of approaching thunderstorms. Yet we have fun here, a lot of fun. We illuminate the upstairs bedroom with a dozen glowing candles in a grand wrought-iron candelabra and listen to old country-style blues recordings on a dented boom box. It's a hot, sweaty August as we swelter under the dentiled eaves, talking like garrulous crows into the thickening velvet nights. Hunter and I laugh ourselves into waves of giddiness, our sides aching and our spirits soaring together. Like two little kids pledging ourselves as best friends forever, we get along like a "house afire," as my grandma Rini would say.

I like this man a lot. Something about him resonates with me. It's a simpatico of sorts. He's intuitive, reading a new situation or a fleeting glance in a millisecond. He lives life by his instincts, following gut hunches and the mood of the day. He leads with his heart, his feelings raw and palpable, coursing off him and into my solar plexus. Ultimately, too, Hunter is a nonconformist. Something wild and wonderful runs through his veins. There are no power plays, ego issues, or ulterior motives between us. We have an honest-to-goodness, clear-cut compat-ibility. Plus my body likes his an awful lot, his flat, sexy stomach sliding against mine, smooth and slick. We cleave to one another in these sultry summer nights.

"Good morning, my goddess," Hunter whispers to me amid the crumpled bedsheets. I smile softly. "I saw an iridescent black form mov-ing in the dark last night," he continues. "At first I thought it was a raven in my dream. Then I blinked and I saw it was you, turning in your sleep. You're bewitching, you know." His kisses flood my skin.

"I am?" I groggily answer.

"Very much so. Like no other."

"Mmmmm…" my voice trails.

"You hold me spellbound. I feel like I've found a long lost part of me in you. You see deep inside my soul with those penetrating dark-brown eyes of yours."

"It's just a looking glass I'm holding up for you," I say. "You see what I know."

Falling in love with Hunter is a christening of sorts to me. I'm born anew, after the nail-sharp misery of these recent years with a crippling illness. My heart grows in the emotional generosity of this thoughtful man. We're true companions of the soul. Often, I'll find my Jeep wheels skittering on the dirt roads as I race through the forest to be by Hunter's side in the quaking months of my marital separation. We visit the sea-shore together, hungering for new horizons and textures. We skinny-dip in hidden lakes at twilight, erasing the torrid heat of the day and the misery from our cells. Hand in hand, Hunter and I forge a brave new path into the world, me as a single mom, he fighting off his daughter's cancer that is once again being monitored closely.

Autumn arrives, bringing with it a full day of school. My dear boy enthusiastically sops up numbers and the alphabet, his small fingers curled tightly on the thick red pencil. He happens to have a knack for math and the gift for gab. I'm overjoyed with all of Eli's new friendships, but transitioning between the two houses can be tough on him at times.

Many nights his softly tendriled words waft around my ears— "Mommy, can I sleep with you?"—as Eli and his beloved stuffed animal crawl up into my big bed. "I'm scared, Mommy. I had a bad dream." Eli burrows himself into my heavy quilts and Peruvian wool blankets as the bitter wind snaps off a branch in a sharp crack.

By Thanksgiving, Joel finally moves out to his own residence. We have bird-nested for five arduous months.

After a run of enormous highs and lows in the months of wrenching apart from Joel, I begin to sense that the sea swells are beginning to taper. Mostly, I'm focused on Eli's well-being, helping him with school and into his new lifestyle of two separate homes. Joel and I agree to joint custody, but that's about all we agree on. Lawyers and mediators fill my life as we pummel our way through financial wranglings. We can agree to nothing. Even the mediators give up in frustration, sending us back to our attorneys.

The divorce process is grueling and harsh. My compass needle is spinning. Some days I have no sense of direction, no sense of self, no sense of my future. It's all I can do to put one foot in front of the other, inching along the rocky facade of a new world. I sell paintings here and there, hoping to get a gallery offer to establish a new career path. One comes in with a small local gallery, boosting my flagging hopes.

Still I sit faithfully at my computer and write my bimonthly health column, which has become an umbilical cord to a sense of normalcy for me. For eighteen years I've been a health-care provider and educator. This vehicle connects me to the constructive parts of me, which I need to remember in this maelstrom. Finances are slipping away. The tail end of my savings can float Eli and me temporarily, but I notice the free-form plummet I'm in and taste the bitter panic in my mouth each morning.

I'm being propelled away from my former life in a seemingly irrational way, running wildly into the headwinds, stretching and reaching for an unknown something. It's an intangible I do not have a name for but can surely feel. I hold on for dear life.

Lull between the Storms

It has already been two years since we lost our dear Echo. I miss her quiet companionship, her ever-present watch over us and the house. Several chickens have vanished in her wake, now more vulnerable to the stalking wildlife.

"When can we get a new puppy?" Eli asks me regularly these days.

"Soon enough, sweetheart. We'll have to find just the right one," I tell him, inwardly uncertain when that might be. I dread the task of housebreaking and obedience training. Plus what kind of dog will be appropriate for just the two of us now? As much as I adore border collies, they need early and careful training. What if Eli and I must move to a smaller space? We'd need a smaller breed.

"We'll keep our eyes open, Eli. Someone will have puppies that need homes," I encourage.

One damp and chilled day, I dash into the old mill building café where I've planned to meet a friend. Rain streaks down the enormous windows, the skies pregnant with a goose-gray light. I scan the cluttered tables for my tall, stunning friend Valerie. Three feet in front of me, my eyes alight on a caramel-and-white bundle of fluff cuddled in Valerie's arms.

"Oh, there you are," she says. "I'm sorry to be late. So many things to distract me."

"Don't worry." I lean in to give her cheek a kiss. "I just arrived, too. But who's this?"

"Oh, our new puppy, Paco. Isn't he adorable?"

"He's more than adorable. He's precious! How old?"

"Just eleven weeks," Valerie tells me. "We got him a few days ago, so I'm hesitant to leave him alone yet. It's all so new for him."

I ask to hold him and she passes the angelic furball to me.

"Oh, my God, Valerie, he's the cutest thing ever." I cuddle the lamb-soft puppy against my neck and shoulder, his wet puppy tongue kissing my face. "He's so dear. What breed is he?"

"Welsh corgi."

I thought he looked familiar! My neighbors had them when I was growing up. They're wonderful dogs. The light goes off in my head. Here's the breed we've been looking for. Valerie gives me the name and website of the breeder.

I'm lit up like a firecracker, eager to tell Eli about today's discovery. Within twenty-four hours I've made contact with Marjorie, the corgi breeder. I ask her a smattering of questions and learn that a new litter is due in a few months. It all sounds good. Excitedly, we await news of Mama Latifah's delivery.

Meanwhile, Joel and I continue to jockey over the divorce process. We are both running on high-octane emotions. Eli often cries now at bedtime. Sarah is living with her mother and has plunged into school-work and dance classes. Blessedly, she still comes to me on Mondays after school for a few hours, enabling us to maintain a connection. I have helped raise her for nine years. From her learning to tie her shoes to reading Dr. Seuss and then into acne, I have loved Sarah. I can't just let her slip away because she's not of my blood. Her soft blue eyes meet mine, confusion and loss, mixed with love and sweetness. I want to see Sarah grow into womanhood. Her fine intelligence and internal strength will propel this pretty girl far in life. My time with Sarah is still needed, and we enjoy our Mondays together.

Life tramps on. Good fortune enables me to study with a portrait master, helping me develop new painting techniques, and I grow to love raw umber. Trying to sell my work, I enter shows and auctions with moderate success. The regional Art Colony studio tour is a major boon for me. I sell eight paintings on the busy, rainy weekend. *Maybe I really can succeed as an artist?*

We move into the holiday season, a note of too much quiet it seems, with my family splintered. On Christmas Eve a loud car horn sounds unexpectedly in our drive. Eli and I run to the door and there stands my dashing father, juggling a tower of wrapped presents.

"Merry Christmas, kids!" he booms, his ever-mischievous smile lit from within. Eli flies into Papou's outstretched arms and tears spring to my eyes.

"This is a wonderful surprise, Daddy!" I exclaim.

"I couldn't bear the two of you being alone, sweetheart," he murmurs into my hair, wrapping me in a bear hug, too.

It's true, the house has a significant void with Joel and Sarah moved out. George's vitality and tickling sprees paint our hearts and holiday with much-needed love and affection.

Hunter moves from the crazy old house into a sweet little apartment in town on a wriggling narrow side street, walking distance to shops and the local pub. Slowly, over the months, Hunter hangs around my place more. He and Eli playfully wrestle and hit baseballs into the fern glade, my son shrieking over Hunter's home-run wallops. He helps me with the house: mowing, raking, shoveling. Hunter's backbone is strong. I cook aromatic meals and Hunter and I dine alfresco, Orion and the Pleiades winking above. How happy we are together.

With the taste of love in my blood, I feel invincible.

Autumnal Equinox

As the months tick by I realize that a full year has passed since the separation. Eli has adapted better than I anticipated. I've grown to know Blue better in this time, too. She comes over with Hunter some days and we do jigsaw puzzles, venture out to yard sales, or play a zany board game called Conga. We surprise Hunter with a homemade, sensationally frosted birthday cake of Blue's personal craftsmanship. From its tenuous beginnings, 2004 is becoming a year of laughter and joy.

Hunter and I decide to take Eli and Blue on a summer vacation into the White Mountains and up to the Maine shore. Along the way we wiggle on our bellies through the dark and snaking Lost River Caves and swim in the frothing rapids of the rushing Swift River. We scream our lungs out, laughing like hyenas, on the Bamboo Chutes ride at Storyland. The last two days of the trip are treasured gems of pristine beauty spent at Hunter's family friend's home, which is tucked neatly into a secluded Maine cove. The children get along famously, trolloping through the mud flats at low tide and slurping up buttered sweet corn and lobster at dinner. We all brave the frigid North Atlantic ocean, dashing in and out of curling waves, tossing the football on shimmering sand. I marvel at the solitude up here on this finger of land jutting out many miles away from civilization.

The salty air is clean and crisp. As the late-day sun dips behind the distant trees, a honeyed glow alights on the sails of an incoming sloop. I think of my youth, the races I skippered and crewed in, relishing the joys of open waters. Now I live inland, shrouded by timberlands and hills. This taste of the shore life reawakens me to the thrill of sea breezes and threatening squalls. At times like this I long for a seaside life, but know within that I chose to move to the highlands for a reason. Life weaves its tapestry.

At the gentlest point of dusk, the evening sky fades to a satiny violet, the sun streaking a final good-bye in tangy hues above the horizon. I watch the sloop make a final tack toward its mooring, the sails luffing momentarily in the turn toward home. Voices lift up off the water, trailing light and garbled on the breeze. At the shoreline, I see Hunter and Blue looking for small sea creatures, bending and rising in their search. I spy Eli roaming amongst the beach plums, plucking out his wayward soccer ball. Ever so quietly, an inner hush caresses my chest. I feel my breathing settle. My mind goes slack and my body relaxes into the deck chair. A moment of deep thanksgiving overtakes me.

We're safe, I think. *There is love.*

I'm here in this place of magnificent wonder, surrounded by new friends, happy children, and a man who loves me. My health is holding. I've rounded a bend.

This still point marks a turning within. Softly, I place my right hand over my heart. Grace and gratitude fill me in this moment of divine presence. I feel profoundly grateful for what I have here in these special people and the magic of their individual spirits. I offer inner thanks to my God force and angels of protection.

Back in Greenvale, September arrives with its cloak of auburn light and sublime weather, wreathing northern New England in the last vestiges of tranquil warmth before the clutch of winter's talons grab hold. Endlessly, I gaze up into the lucid blue sky, marveling at just how glorious this month of the year is. The air stands still with mere traces of feather-soft breezes swaying the fading bee balm and lush periwinkle asters on their tall stems. Dragonflies dart about on parade, while apples hang ripe and thick from the craggy orchard trees behind the fern-trimmed stone wall. Eli, Sarah, and I gather the darkest red ones to bake into a pie.

Early autumn is so rich in its harvest, lushly laden with earthen smells, textured in the changing tones. I run high on the heady elixir of such sensual bounty, sopping up each day with its lustrous glory. The back-to-school routine settles in. Eli's in second grade now. A strong-shouldered teenage boy comes two times a week to stack wood for me, rake leaves, turn over the garden, and ready us for winter. I've begun job hunting, sending out resumes, filling out applications, looking for some steady work. Nothing has surfaced yet, though. Maintaining this house with two mortgages, taxes, upkeep, and no child support costs me a lot. Scarcity is the norm. Tension grips me too tightly these days.

I try to see a few former homeopathic clients, in an effort to once more test the waters. It's hard work and my once laser-fine memory is now fuzzy. My head aches from only two hours of thinking. It's weird to discover that I may not be as healthy as I thought I was. Once considered a talented homeopath, I now fumble through my repertory and materia medica. Something inside me is actually recoiling at the idea of caring for other people's problems, which comes as a shock to me. My energy is disappointingly rather sketchy again as of late. I notice a nosedive in the afternoon. If I close my eyes to rest, I fall into a sudden sleep.

I am caught off guard and somewhat disturbed by the fact that the robust health I experienced over the past eighteen months is waning. This weary afternoon flag and the sweaty nighttime sleep are too reminiscent of my sickly past. *Please let this be just a minuscule dip,* I pray, propping up my homeopathic remedy and vitamin arsenal yet again.

Up on the Moors

T he clanging of the harbor bell rings with a clarion shrill through the thickening milky fog. I bundle deeper into my plaid woolen muffler, gingerly wrapping my stiff and pained neck. Ever so carefully, I baffle strained muscles with just the right degree of pressure from the scarf, struggling to deter the piercing Nantucket wind straight off the darkening ocean. Damp and raw, it pries viciously on my sensitive skin.

The "wind gates" is what the old Chinese physicians call this tender spot on the back of one's neck. Winter's creeping dampness can be trapped there as it drives its way into the body at this precarious spot. Then inflammation sets in, the influenza brews, or the sniffles emerge as the body vies to purge the winds. I honor this wisdom and bundle up some more, out on the remote reaches of Nantucket.

I love Nantucket. To me, it's a place of haunting passages. It feels like I walk between the veils of the worlds out here on this oceanic island. All of it—the stretching beach sands, the romantic heather moors, the cobbled whaling village streets—throws me back in time, propelling me into a déjà vu sensation. In fact, I often wrestle with my conscious mind out here. Yesterday in town, I fleetingly saw what I thought was the half-turned face of my father; he was cloaked in a jet-black, collared cape and top hat.

No, I reminded myself. *He's back home in his house on the Hudson River, not here at an oaken desk, behind a leaded-glass window.* It was eerie to have seen him inside that storefront. *You're daydreaming, Kim.*

Images waver in and out of my mind's eye regularly on this polka dot of island terrain, though. Whenever I visit Nantucket, time shimmers and melts before me, messages blowing through my thoughts the way the wind does in my neck, impressing wisdom and warnings alike. Scenes appear before me, ghostlike, as I tramp along sandy footpaths or bike out to the shoals. The gleanings are gripping and visceral in their emotional footprint, colorful and textured with feelings and even history. My mother called them "picture stories" when I told her of them as a child.

"Your grandma Rini had them too, dear. But please, Kim, do not pry into other people's lives with this vision of yours. They deserve their own privacy," she warned and scared me simultaneously. By my teens, I learned to shut the "picture stories" down.

In this early October of 2004, I've come to Nantucket with Hunter on a painting commission. My assignment is to capture four landscape scenes of a family's beloved heirloom of land and cottage, situated sweetly on a tucked away lee of the rambling heather moors. It's one of the few old-style properties left on the island, understated in its simplicity and scrimshaw charm. The two-bedroom house, tiny in dimension yet raftered with family memories floating off the pages of the guest book, reminds me of my own barefooted childhood gambols collecting sand dollars and jingle shells along the still uncluttered shores of Fire Island and Martha's Vineyard.

I head out, laden with paints and canvases, portable easel in tow, hiking up and down the moorland swales, searching and finding a nice pinnacle from which to paint. The amber Indian summer light bathes the endless swaths of russet-and-sienna heathers in breathtaking beauty. It's actually quite daunting to try to portray the sensual beauty of these moors. I wrestle with two canvases well into the final weeping indigo rays of evening's surrender. The next day I'm back again, tangled in my own attempts to capture the moors on my canvases.

By noon I'm drenched in sweat and paints, half-clothed, and simultaneously euphoric and distraught, moved by the solitude and majesty of this untouched land, yet displeased with my efforts. The paintings are not as delicate as I had aimed for. Instead, they're marked by broad strokes and even broader colors. *Oh, well,* I think, *tomorrow I'll paint the ocean instead.* Unfortunately, while I trudge back to the cottage, a splitting headache and stiff neck mount rapidly.

By late afternoon I'm cramped in the vise of a wicked migraine. It holds siege throughout the next day, which is shrouded in mists and a drizzling, raw rain. Hunter helps me ride out my pain with ice packs and meds.

By evening, I'm still sick. Hunter and I struggle unsuccessfully to get the CD player to work. The ocean wind, murmuring in the shrunken pines at our window's edge, traces a haunting song into my soul, sending me deeper into the trancelike state of Nantucket's magic. Even though the pine song is lovely, we both sorely want to hear a favorite CD of ours. The player works for a line or two, then jams up. We have fussed with it for hours in frustration.

The headache has plastered me down pretty badly. Being a migraineur of two decades I can categorize them all by various self-standards. This one is particularly fierce, zapping my energy, making my mind foggy, and leaving me feeling dizzy and fragile. Thirty-six hours into it, even on the usually effective medication, I'm waiting out the passing of the final stages of the siege. I lie in a zombie posture on the denim-blue sofa, watching the candle flame flicker and listening to Hunter clatter pots and pans in the kitchen. I study the woodworking inlays of the cathedral ceiling, noticing shapes and faces hidden in the whitewashed knotty pine. This time span of waiting and studying my environs in stillness and scrutiny is not unusual for me—rather, a familiar place of my life that I visit periodically while moving through the ravages of a migraine. It is odd to acknowledge that the migraines have taught me how to become an acutely sensitive observer of my environment. In many ways they have actually accentuated my razor-fine skill of observation.

Essentially, this is a happy experience here on the island in spite of the migraine and weather. Hunter and I are blissfully content alone together, reveling in the romantic solitude of this idyllic setting. We chat and loll, nibble on savories, he plowing through a novel. Outside the window we watch flocks of goldfinches dangling from the bushes and branches, gobbling up the shiny autumn berries. Out of the blue I get an urge to telephone my mother and tell her about the beauty of this place, for a moment having forgotten that she died seven years ago. I see an image of her in my mind's eye, her soft brown hair and brilliant smile. I begin to quietly cry, tears trickling down my cheeks. Suddenly, it's almost like I feel her hand brush my brow, tucking my matching brown hair behind my ear.

Hunter, ever intuitive, walks out from the kitchen, asking me, "What's wrong?"

"How did you know?" I reply, tears pouring.

"I felt a cold chill go down my spine and a sense that someone was standing beside me at the stove," he says. "And then this pull inside me to come check on you."

It's uncanny how aligned he and I are.

He sits down next to me, teetering on the sofa's edge while drying his hands on the terry-cloth dish towel. "Why are you crying, honey?"

"I felt my mother," I whimper. "I think she's here."

"I think that was her in the kitchen, too," he says.

With that I cry more. Hunter cradles me in his arms and rocks me. I miss my mother so much. She was my steady beacon. Gentle, nurturing, patient, and understanding, always able to corral my reckless energy into a tempered and more appropriate direction. My father and sister claim they sense her presence regularly. Me, never. I feel she's been gone from me physically and spiritually for a very long time.

Hunter and I sit together in silence, he holding my hand.

"Can I see if we can talk to her?" I suggest to Hunter. "Let's see if she can make herself known to us. If she's really here."

Hunter looks at me a bit skeptically, being more sensibly earthbound than I, but he doesn't say no.

I try to imagine what exactly I should say to welcome my mother. Finally, I just say a few words that pop into my mind.

"Mother, thank you for coming here. I miss you so much. Life's so different without you. You've never met my gorgeous son, Eli. Oh, how you would adore him. But I'm very grateful you can reach me like this out here on the moors. We both feel you, we think." I sniffle a little more. "Mother, if you're really here, can you please prove it to us by making something known to us here in the cottage? Some sort of evidence?"

Hunter is stock-still. I know he thinks I'm nuts.

"How about this?" I say. "Can you make the CD player work so we can listen to Dido? It's been broken and the CD has a lot of special meaning to us."

I see Hunter squinting at me.

"Go on, turn it on," I urge him.

He gets up and turns on the CD player. It starts up as it has before. It plays the now familiar two lines of music, then plays the whole CD through without stopping! For over thirty-five minutes we listen to the music. At the very end of the last song, it stops only one line from the finish. No matter how we rattle and shake it, pressing buttons and knobs in earnest, it won't play again.

We're impressed, a tad shivery, and certainly fairly shocked. I'm touched at a very core level. Apparently this is a visitation, something neither of us has experienced before. It seems to hold us in a half-kilter place of both belief and disbelief. We sit motionless, staring at one another for the next half hour, speechless, afraid to shift the energies, and questioning our sense of reality.

I go to sleep that night with an internal running conversation streaming toward the spirit form of my mother. It's stunning and a precious gift to have felt a connection with her. I'm awed and hear a trailing voice in my mind, "Stay strong and believe in yourself, no matter what, Kim!" The sentence runs over and over, in a rumbling tone of a locomotive engine, boring firmly into my being. This, I trust, is a message from Mother.

The next day dawns, heavily mired in more fog. The headache lingers, though not as bad. It remains well into my final day here. I force myself to work on the commissions, sketching now, since the light is so poor. I feel incredibly weak, though, with barely enough energy to walk down the drive and back. I'm unable to venture back up onto the moorland hills.

I lumber home to New Hampshire, dazed and not well. The Nantucket experience lays a muzzy film on me.

Getting Lucky

Marjorie, the corgi breeder, emails to say that a beautiful litter has arrived. Mother and pups are all in excellent health. There are six boys and five girls, and she wants to know which we prefer.

"Just pick us out the mellowest one in the group," I write back. "Temperament is most important."

"Sure enough, darlin'."

We check in periodically and Marjorie kindly keeps us abreast of the puppies' progress. We chat on the phone, confirming that she's watching to see who will develop into a "relaxed" dog. Our excitement mounts. Soon enough Marjorie sends us photos of three puppies she considers to be good choices for us.

"They're all sweet as peaches 'n' cream. Two are girls and one is a boy. Why don't y'all look at these pictures and let me know which puppy y'all like the best. Then we can compare notes."

Anyone would melt over the cuteness quotient of these dewy-eyed pups. I happen to prefer the caramel-and-white one, but say nothing of this to Eli when he comes home from school later in the day.

"Sweetheart, look at these pictures and tell me which puppy you'd choose for us," I tell Eli.

He handily selects the same one as me. That evening when he comes over for dinner, I show the photos to Hunter.

"Which puppy do you like for us? We don't know which one Marjorie has earmarked. She's going to tell us after we're done with our selection."

He looks them over, sitting at the swivel stool at my kitchen counter.

"This one," he says, showing me the very same photo that Eli and I have chosen.

"Why that one?"

"I like his eyes. They're sensitive. Plus I think the coat is the thickest of the three. It looks lush."

"Well, we've each picked the same puppy!" I say, grinning in pleasure. "I'll call Marjorie."

A few minutes later I'm speaking to Tennessee. "Marjorie, which pup did you select for us?"

"Oh, darlin', I think the little fellow in picture number three is just a lamb. He's the sweetest darn thing. A bit shy and not as feisty as his two sisters. I been watchin' them all closely the past few days and even though he's a male and you'd think he'd tend to be more aggressive and rough, he's not. He's bigger than the girls, but just so sweet and more mellow. In fact, I scolded him this mornin' for peein' on the floor, and, darlin', he just had the saddest, most hurt look on his face. What a little doll."

I'm giving Eli and Hunter the thumbs-up sign, grinning as I speak into the receiver.

"Well, Marjorie, that's who we all picked, too. That's just perfect." I practically scream in excitement. We go over the details of vaccinations, payment, and the puppy's shipping plans. He'll be traveling to us on US Air, with a plane transfer in Philly.

"He'll be in his own carrier, hon, with a soft blanket and a stuffed toy animal of his own. He'll travel with water, but I don't give 'em medication. They do just fine this way. Believe me, we've done it many times now. Y'all just hold him and love him when y'all pick him up and he'll be fine."

Eli and I mark the calendar with our puppy's arrival date, October 13, and start the anxious countdown. Finally, it arrives. We're so excited. I pick Eli up from school and we make the hour drive east to the closest commercial airport. Hunter is planning to meet us there. Eli and I slip through the sliding glass doors, entering the arrival area bustling with travelers. Upon scanning the overhead flight information screens, my heart drops in dismay. The puppy's plane will be delayed for two hours. Our balloon of jubilation deflates. We must kill time in the airport, torture for an active and eager eight-year-old.

While standing upstairs in the observation tower, leaning against the wooden handrail and watching planes take off and land, I feel a sudden discomforting wave of vertigo. The floor before me spins and I must sit down on a nearby bench. Over the next hour, as Eli energetically scampers up and down the stairs and squirms on the deep windowsill, I feel an awful weakness and fatigue descending on me, like a heavy, ancient tapestry curtain. A slightly queasy stomach bothers me. Hunter notices my wan complexion and keeps a protective eye on both me and my son.

"Sit down, honey. You look tired," he says.

I nod and mechanically do as instructed.

Finally, the long-overdue flight arrives. By now the sky has darkened to pitch. We watch the plane taxi to the gate, its running lights twinkling in the sea of darkness. Eli studies the men on the tarmac signaling the aircraft in with handheld lights and gyrating arm gestures. He then leads the pack as we get ourselves quickly back downstairs to the baggage claim area and our puppy's arrival destination.

After what feels like an incredibly long thirty minutes, with all the passenger suitcases having been collected, a thin man in a navy-blue jumpsuit walks out a side door with a pet carrier in his hands. We circle toward him. Inside is the most precious ball of butterscotch-and-white down imaginable. As we open the latched door, a warm, soft, wiggling bundle of beauty climbs into my arms, his tongue licking me in instant happiness. We are in love.

Eli and I can't stop hugging our new puppy. We pass him back and forth between our arms. We're told that he hasn't eaten, but the personnel in Philly did take him out to pee. We find some Milk-Bones in my pocket and Eli watches over him like a seasoned mother hen while Hunter and I settle up the paperwork. Then, home we go, the puppy nestled on Eli's lap, me blearily pointing the Jeep westward.

"Lucky, Mommy, let's call him Lucky!" Eli says gleefully on our trek home.

"Sounds like a winner to me," I tell him, with a smile.

With the way I feel, though, we're going to need more than luck.

Crashing

The ensuing months of autumn become a living nightmare. The curtain of weakness that descended in the observation tower never lifts. Dizzy spells come and go. In the usual busy season of autumn winterization—garden cleanup, wood stacking, and vegetable canning—I'm suddenly incapacitated. I get Eli off to school each day, then crash. Days are slipping away from me. Nothing is getting done. I can't even look for a job. I'm floored by the exhaustion and relentless migraines that began in Nantucket. My head is in a constant fog, my gut a wreck. I'm plastered on the sofa, barely able even to let the puppy out for housebreaking. I note a bruised feeling all over my body. Plus there's this thready kind of predawn insomnia. My doctor and neurologist both run batteries of tests, scopes, and scans. I drink barium; I'm injected with dyes. Still, I feel like hell, like I'm breaking apart. Labs return: no Epstein-Barr, no Lyme disease, no thyroid disease.

Suddenly, a suspect scan comes in, highlighting a glowing tumor on my right kidney. I'm catapulted into a kidney specialist's office at Dartmouth Hospital, with an oncologist and French-accented surgeon awaiting my arrival. I sit there in shock as I'm examined, listening to the oncologist's recommendation.

"This is considered a tiny tumor. It isn't causing any of these systemic symptoms. Let's wait and watch you for six months. However," he cautions, "it could be serious. Don't neglect this."

I nod yes, now in a state of emotional trauma. A follow-up appointment is scheduled for May. Hunter wheelchairs me to the car. I cry the entire ninety-minute ride home. Terror roars through my pysche.

I crash at home, propped up on my tranquilizers, and feel as stunned as a bird who has hit a window. I'm too weak to drive, sleep is raggedy, and my head spins. My blood sugar feels like it's constantly plummeting; I feel jittery and starving, and have anxiety rushes that only a solid protein meal can assuage. My metabolism has gone way out of whack. Suddenly, I'm packing on weight in a way I never have before.

I keep harping to the doctors that something is ransacking my chemistry. "Check my thyroid, my adrenals, my pancreas," I beseech.

I lean heavily on my trusted homeopath, Melinda, in Massachusetts, to balance me. The homeopathic remedies at least settle my nerves and help me sleep solidly.

Days run into nights, nights into days, with me falling down a dark elevator shaft of despair. Joel helps out by keeping Eli an extra night on weekends. Poor Hunter is now cooking, doing laundry, and toting my kids about, while commuting to work sixty minutes away. I'm basically incapacitated. The intensity bores in even more dramatically than four years ago. I'm scared beyond words.

I'm racked with a weird vibrating feeling in my body and a high-pitched buzz in my head. No one else can hear it when I quiz them. Burning, knifelike stomach pains, bloaty, gassy expansions, and bizarre 3 a.m. ravenous hunger pangs are intense. My GI tract is a mess. After the scans and cultures and blood tests mount, all that can be determined is that I have some mild digestive flora deficiencies and perhaps a pH imbalance leaning toward the acidic.

"Everything else is fine, Kim," Malcolm, my new GP, and the experts proclaim.

I'm confused by these medical explorations. Suspecting a malfunction in my gut, I end up following my own instincts and holistic understandings, and attempt to soothe these persistent discomforts on my own.

Since I'm too weak to climb the stairs unassisted, Hunter guides me up from behind, holding my hips for balance and a boost. We navigate around the oaken newel post at the left of the landing, steering toward the bedroom. In Hunter's right hand he holds my bedtime tray, a train of ducklings strung single file across its edge. It's absurd that this former wedding gift, anointing a glorious occasion, now houses the poultices for my pained and ornery tummy.

Graham crackers, a banana, a small yogurt, probiotic capsules, and ginger tea faithfully make their way to my bedside table. I nibble on the crackers, down my tablets, and sip my tea as Eli and puppy Lucky clamor on board for bedtime books. My head feels heavy lidded, obtuse, and waterlogged. With trembling hands I turn the pages of *Go, Dog. Go!* Eli and I nestle together, his stuffed animal and Lucky between us, as I weave through the twenty-one pages once again. In these blissful moments I swallow hard. This is my one spell of comfort in the long slavish days of illness.

Why can't the doctors give me any answers other than a suspect virus? Oh, how I wish my mother were alive. She'd help me, heal me, find me the proper health care. All I have of her are the mystical words that wafted in on the haunting spell of the Nantucket's moors. "Stay strong and believe in yourself, no matter what, Kim."

Christmas Day is surreal to me. Eli and Blue are sensationally enthused to discover Santa's offerings. I can barely sit upright for thirty minutes in the down-cushioned armchair. My limbs are quaking, my pulse erratic, my head packed with cotton. I recall nothing other than the sound of childhood jubilance and the crinkling tear of wrapping paper.

By the next morning Hunter has me in the ER. I can't stop trembling and am so weak I can't stand. He half carries me from the car. Waiting forever on the rigid gurney, it feels like I'm evaporating into some distant place.

Another exam. More blood tests. Waiting, waiting, waiting.

The ER doctor says that everything looks normal.

"Then why am I so weak?" I implore.

"It's most likely a mysterious virus."

I've heard that one before. "Is my SED rate high or are my WBCs off?"

"No, nothing's irregular." He shakes his head and tells me just to get some rest. "The holidays may have drained you."

"But I've been sick since October and getting worse. My head and eyes feel like they're layered in gauze."

He just shakes his head, at a loss for an explanation.

We go home and I cry some more. No one knows how to help me. I'm angry and frustrated by our supposedly capable medical system. I feel so let down and betrayed. In the past three months I've disinte-grated rapidly. I've devoted twenty years to healing others; why can't someone help me?

The next day Hunter bumps into our yoga instructor in town. While he's recounting how stricken I am with an undiagnosable condition, she instantaneously blurts out to him, "Dr. Wu! She's a master acupuncturist and most surely will help Kim."

We attain an appointment by week's end.

Dr. Wu turns out to be a gifted, kind, intuitive, and amazingly pro-ficient acupuncturist and Chinese herbalist. She literally takes me by the hand and helps me take my first few steps out of this well of darkness.

"Liver tight. Stomach cold. Kidney chi low. Emotions too big," Dr. Wu pronounces on taking my pulses. "Must eat only cooked food, noth-ing raw. Even fruit must be cooked. Ginger tea a lot."

I follow her orders and additionally down some bitter herbal con-coction she gives me. As many herbals as I've taken in my twenty-plus years in natural medicine, I must say this is one of the most wicked of them all. I find myself nearly retching as the crumbling dry leaves and twigs inch down my throat. I swallow a spoonful of honey to fend off the aftertaste.

Hunter and some of my friends juggle transporting me to and from this third-generation Chinese physician. She's knowledgeable and com-petent, undeterred by my state.

"You get well," she confidently tells me, patting my hand during another teary bout.

The snows pound hard, icy roads loom, and we still make the bi-weekly trek to her office. I'm propped on pillows, the passenger seat fully reclined in an attempt to reduce my nausea and weakness. Sadly, during this time of trial, I have finally had to give up the newspaper health column. It is just too hard to do. For a couple of months I wrote out the articles in longhand and Hunter or Charlene would type them. Now, my mind is too shot even to focus on a topic or the research. Tragically, it feels as if my entire career has swirled down the drain. It is a crushing loss for me, a wound gripping my heart.

About six weeks into treatment I start to feel a lift in my state. My head is becoming less fog-filled, and I actually find a window of improved energy in late morning. I force myself to take Lucky out for a daily walk, up and around the circle. Convinced that fresh air and movement will help, I wrap my scarf and hat tightly as we trudge through the penetrating winds of winter. Then, back indoors, I collapse on the bed.

Hunter and I have taken to a new routine during these weeks. When Eli is at his father's home, I stay with Hunter in his tiny but convenient apartment in town. I feel less isolated there than alone all day in my woodland home. It has a sunny living room and kitchen, cheerful with white-stained wooden floors and red-gingham wallpaper. The chatter of voices as people pass on the sidewalk outside lifts my spirit. Hunter leaves for work in the morning, having pre-made a tuna sandwich and set aside juice and snacks for me. I can barely manage the dozen or so steps to the bathroom or kitchen from the bed. I'm tenaciously hanging on, as insecurity soils my consciousness. I listen to John Lee Hooker again and again on the stereo, his mahogany voice crooning blues refrains into my being.

"Milk and alcohol soothe my nerves," he warbles. I relate to the crying strain of his voice, the misery of a broken man's life mirroring my own in this raw song of suffering.

I become intimately familiar with the arc of the sun, watching its cast move across the room and sky in the span of my days here on Ivy Street. It rises cool and blue-flanged on the sloping snowbanks of the driveway across the street. I watch the weathered charcoal planking of the neighbor's teetering nineteenth-century shed meld from umber to ash as the sunlight plays on its south and west walls. By day's end shadows stretch flat and long from a low-slung cloud front. The bare, flutelike branches of the sturdy trees shiver in the fierce Canadian-blown winds.

Will I ever recover? I feel so alone, trapped inside these walls of myself in the vicious clutches of this endless illness. Still, small gestures warm my heart in big proportions. Hunter and I eat our dinners in front of the TV, guffawing hilariously at old reruns of *Seinfeld*. I laugh out loud, noting the rush of happiness filling my chest. Eli and I discover that back-gammon comes easily to him. We play game after game, outstretched on my bed or on the cozy living room sofa. Sure enough, when Eli once again defeats me, laughter fills my lungs with gleeful expansion.

"I won!" my wide-eyed child crows.

I beam with pride.

My dear Welsh corgi puppy has taken on stuffed animal qualities of comfort. When my fears or sadness become too engulfing, I lift the soft bundle of fur into my arms, and we lie snuggled together, his toasty body placed right up against my trembling heart. Soon enough a glow-ing presence of love fills me, easing away the crowding sphere of inter-nal discomfort. Thump-thump, thump-thump, I feel our hearts beating together. A joyful puppy lick, and again I hear my own laughter.

Baby steps, I keep telling myself. *Each day is a baby step of progress. Each stride forward is movement in the right direction. I'm here, no worse, not back-sliding, feeling some minuscule droplets of hope.*

The Glades

Dr. Wu drops me to one visit per week, which is a positive sign. Eli and I ready ourselves for our annual trip to sunny Fort Lauderdale. Will I have the stamina to endure travel? On trembling legs at baggage pickup, I fear I might just fall to the ground, but willpower guides me out the sliding doors, into a cab, and home to my father's elegant condo in the sky.

The streaming Florida sun infuses me with volumes of healing energy. Lying flat on the warmed, powdery sand, I sense the earth below me. I want nothing more than to lie here by the hour, drawing out the impurities of whatever microbe has invaded me. Somehow I always regain my vitality after days on the beach. Eli returns north and I take in another week. By the time Hunter arrives for a few days of R&R, he's elated to find me smiling, suntanned, and visibly upright at the front door.

"Honey, you look terrific!" he says, wrapping me in a big hug.

"I'm doing better." I grin proudly. "The weather's been perfect."

On a lark, three days later we decide to go out to the Everglades to show Hunter the natural beauty, tall grasses swaying in this rich effluvial marsh. South Florida is my second home, since much of my family has resided here since the early 1940s. Childhood memories brim with coots and anhingas, slashing open coconuts in the yard, or counting gators in the ditchwater canals abutting the old cement roads. My grandparents operated the local bar and package store in downtown Homestead, Florida. With twin-talking mynah birds and the flyboys from the air force base littering the long lacquered bar, their place held a smoky mystery to us grandkids in the 1960s. All these years later, I want to see if it is possible to find a piece of the untamed Old Florida, from the time before the shopping plaza grid and high-rise courtship choked off its native charms.

Loping my dad's '73 Buick off the road onto a sandy lane, Hunter and I find a small airboat concession, a ramshackle hut glaring in the midday sun. The weathered captain takes us on a hair-raising ride, fish-tailing the flat-bottomed boat on wide-banked turns, the water spraying in huge arcs. The delicate marsh grasses shimmy and part as we side-slip through the endless twisting river, the engine blaring ferociously behind us. The remarkable thing is that on this exhilarating, high-speed adventure, I notice my energy shifting dramatically from murky malaise to a clearer, higher vibration. Somehow, by expanding into the speed and freedom, I've rattled free from the clutches of fear and depression. I am enlivened in a powerful way!

We alight back on land, me light-headed and buzzing in the rush of the intoxicating excursion. Walking toward the Buick I'm aware that this sensation I'm feeling is none other than euphoria. I'm riding a tremendous neurochemical surge and it feels good! Rolling down the car windows, I realize we are not far from dear old Homestead and coax Hunter into taking a spin to my old stomping grounds.

Soon enough we roll into town. I readily recognize my grandparents' former home, still sturdy and strong, but remodeled from its 1920s origins. The terra-cotta roof, the angle of the March sunlight, and spacious avocado trees throw me back in time as I step onto the familiar, pocked limestone sidewalk. Sleeping memories awaken: my mother's girlish laughter, fresh laundry on the line, Grandpa's curling pipe smoke. I bend down, touching the sandy earth, the footprints of my past, and many feel-good moments of my youth. It's a touchstone of my durable roots. As we climb back in the Buick, I turn for one last glimpse at our homestead. Tears of fondness gather in my eyes.

Searching for the bar, we make all the correct turns, and there it is on the old railroad tracks, now more shadowed amid an outcropping of newer buildings, but still a downtown working-class bar. I open the heavy, metal door and enter the dark interior. Soaking in the ambience, I sit in disbelief. So little has changed. The same signed Elvis photo, the neon Seagram's sign, my grandfather's velvet Shriners hat, and the patinaed brass beer taps of thirty-five years ago are all in their identical spots. I feel like I'm in a time warp. This has been quite a day.

Laying my head on my pillow at bedtime, emotions and new currents of energy course through me. Curling up close to Hunter, I know I've unleashed a grip that clamped me tight. I'm infusing myself with the ability to move ahead. I can let go of my past, recurrent illness included.

When I get back to New Hampshire, I decide, I'm going to put my house on the market. I'll find a sunny little place to rent in town, and make a fresh start.

Sleep comes quickly.

Prep Time

Back home in New Hampshire my energy isn't great, but it's enough to bolster me in my determination to sell the house. I am able to spend an hour or so each morning cleaning out closets, drawers, and storage areas, making the place more appealing to sell. Hunter works like a demon and finishes laying a new roof on the barn. A big yard sale removes much excess from my dwelling. By late May, though, my energy begins to bottom out again.

In June 2005 the house is listed with a prestigious realty firm. Early swells of summer fill the yard with generous green trees and my poppies blooming in a particularly high bonanza of crimson glory.

Now let the perfect buyer manifest! I pray for someone secure, with easy financing, not dependent on a prior house selling, and ready to close by September. I write these criteria on a wish list and place it on my bathroom mirror, daily willing the future buyer to me. The realtors start showing the house promptly. My hopes are high.

A week later, though, I feel something is definitely going terribly awry in me again. While sitting in the bleachers at one of Eli's Little League games, I note my heart is skipping beats and my stomach feels queasy. My energy starts to plummet. By nightfall I'm flat on the sofa again, my head feeling cloudy and heavy, my limbs leaden, and my chest hollow. Hunter says my color has drained. Over the next two weeks I sink deeper and deeper into an awful funnel of downward energy, which overwhelms me, along with depression and a molasses malaise.

I enter my doctor's office, tear-strewn and scared. "It's back," I tell him. "The whole situation from last winter has returned in full force. Now the anxiety waves and migraines are setting in, too." I feel desperate and frantic. Something is seriously wrong with me.

Dr. Pennell examines me, assessing a sinus infection and most likely a viral component. As usual, blood tests and scans are ordered. I wait and pray at home. For five years now I've been moving in and out of these collapses, with no true healing, merely episodes of relief. It's time for the kidney tumor follow-up, too, but I am so weak, so weak that I can't even stand up, that I must postpone this necessary test. I am wretchedly, appallingly ill.

Once again I telephone my homeopath in Massachusetts. Hunter drives me down for an appointment a week later. Despite all the testing from Dr. Pennell, I show no clinical findings.

"These are subclinical symptoms," Melinda tells me. "No pathology has set in, which indicates that you're afflicted with a 'syndrome,' like chronic fatigue syndrome. You yourself know homeopathy can correct such an imbalance."

"Doctor heal thyself, huh?" I joke. The irony isn't lost on either of us.

"I'm behind you," she promises. "We'll find your remedy, Kim. Hang in there. Let me email Jayesh for his help." She gives me a big, warm, sympathetic hug.

In the days that follow, a heat wave mounts with cloying thickness, swaddling us in tropical air masses blown north to our granite-ridged highlands. Daily I force myself off the sofa and, dangling on Hunter's right arm, attempt a walk around the perimeter of my backyard. In all honesty, twenty-five steps is a huge endeavor, my lungs weakly straining in the humidity, my limbs quivering. Some days we cut the passage short, me collapsing back on the couch amid tears of despair.

I'm downing vitamins and herbs by the handful to boost my immune system. The trusted homeopathic remedy that Melinda prescribes guides me through draining the sinus infection and clearing up the cotton head. Friends cart me to and from the acupuncturists' and Reiki practitioners' offices. My GP tenderly encourages me to hold on, saying that I can overcome this derailment. His findings once again show notable elevated EBV titres; he thinks it's a reactivated infection.

"You need not to overdo it, Kim. Please lay low for six weeks."

The words are miserable to my ears. "I need to sell my house," I protest.

"Rest, Kim. We have to protect your spleen."

Blessedly, the realtors only bring two or three customers by to see my home over the critical weeks I lie helplessly collapsed and dejected, once again watching gorgeous summer days fly by outside my windows. It's a scene now all too forlornly familiar. The summer creaks onward.

Eagle's Wings

Ilie flat as a railway bed for month after month, throughout the humid summer of 2005. Too weak to lift my head for more than a few minutes at a time, I manage being vertical for only the most directed necessities: a trip to the bathroom, sitting up to eat, changing my clothes. As dawn breaks, Hunter stirs me from under my heavy, sodden sleep with a breakfast tray of eggs, juice, and toast. Eli, in his eight-year-old zest, crawls atop my bed for a pre-camp kiss, then flits out the door for his freewheeling day.

The air conditioners drone, the house lies still, like a lion lounging in the heat of the African plains. Outside the silent windows, I see the sun blazing, the hollyhocks climbing, the heat mounting. All I can manage is a rotation of position, from left side to right and then over supine onto my back. Faithfully, each day, I force myself out of my bed and pajamas. If I linger too long in either, my spirits flag so deeply into a plummeting trench of despair and fear that it's close to impossible to fathom a return to wellness. Months into this recent nosedive, I'm self-trained to avoid emotional or psychic influences triggering deepening depression.

I slide down the stairs, propping myself on the oak handrail, diving directly onto the waiting sofa, managing to flick on the CD player en route. The same five discs have been playing round and round for two months now, daily. Hours on end, the chords and harmonies waft around my cotton-filled head. I've ascertained that these are just the right sounds to soothe my jangled nerves and trembling limbs. I answer no phones, look at no TV, turn on no computers, read nothing. I'm in a vacuum, detached from the world, its bustling societal activities, political happenings, and even trends in the weather. All day, alone and motionless, I wrestle instead with my own seismic quakes and shifts. I can handle nothing more.

I proclaim myself a hothouse plant, as any minor external fluctuation can send me into a completely disharmonious flux. Direct sunlight, a five-degree temperature shift, the air conditioner drafting on me, the wrong pillow, a slamming door are all aggravators. I hate it. I'm beyond catlike finicky. I feel as if I've been taken hostage by my malingering body. It blows my mind. Formerly vital, spontaneous, and even reckless, now I'm in a state of captive restraint and stillness.

I've never before known how to be this still. I've been studying the same twelve maple leaves out the window for weeks now. I start to think about loneliness and death and the possibility of true miracles. In these decaying times I become acquainted with parts of myself I never knew existed. It's as if I'm discovering a piece of terrain in the vast tableau of the universe in which I occupy less than a nanosecond of importance. These conceptual facts feel daunting and spectral in a sense. My insignificance begins to take precedence in my thought patterns. Who am I really? Why am I even here?

I cry a lot, long, heaving sobs that clench my stomach muscles. At night, I cry quiet, self-pitying tears, drowning in the abyss of my own unknown—the unknown of this illness, of my future, of my conscious and unconscious minds. A part of me is close to giving up hope. But I cling desperately to a very tiny flicker of inner knowing that I will not give up. Having spent so much of my life in natural medicine, I deeply trust there are ways, maybe yet unclear to me, that will help my body right itself and start to heal. I refuse to give up on that belief.

I rummage through my thoughts and feelings, thinking of so many novels and poems cataloguing deaths resulting from sadness. The despair, the depression, the overwhelming grief within breaks these characters' beings, their will, their ability to breathe and live in a normal sense. They die. I have seen the elderly lose hope and die after the death of a beloved spouse. To die from sadness.

Will I, too, die now? Am I literally dying? Some days I grapple with this notion. Is this a terminal illness? Is it a disease not yet captured on film or lab testing? These numbing limbs and flopping feet feel like MS in a way. Maybe Lou Gehrig's disease? But the neurologist at Dartmouth has confirmed that I have no neurological disease process. The kidney specialist and oncologists say I do not have a cancer. The internists say that my GI trouble is irritable bowel syndrome and that the Esptein-Barr titres are once again high. But why? Thousands of dollars later, scans and scopes infinitum, I lie pallid and inert, like a lifeless brook trout no longer even able to flail or flop a silvery fin. There is nothing more to do but to rest and wait, take my vitamins and homeopathic remedies, see the acupuncturist. I pray…but I'm close to giving up.

I call my father, wailing into the phone. "I'm so weak. I don't think I'll ever get well."

My eternally optimistic, strong to the very marrow of the soul father will not let me give up. Having fought back from three near-death experiences, white light and all, during his eighty years on earth, he gives me another of his famous pep talks.

"You can do it, Kim. Hang in there. You're strong, very strong. Don't forget you are a Makris. We're tough, Black Sea Greeks. There's nothing you can't overcome. Use your will, sweetheart. Use your will. Think of a beautiful place you love. Use it as a way to soothe your mind. Don't forget you have a young son you need to raise and be there for. No one but you can give him the tender, loving care that only you so perfectly know how to show. Please, sweetheart, know that you can do this. Be patient. Look at all that I beat out, even when they told me I would die!"

I continue to whimper, but I listen to him, as I always have when in trouble. My father is right, always right about the big things in life. He's a stunning man, gifted with so much wisdom, integrity, and a will of proportions rarely glimpsed in life. Having been left to die in the trenches of the Philippines in WWII, he was found by medics days later and managed to rally from a broken back, shrapnel blinding one eye, crystallized kidneys, and more. In my youth, I saw him beat encephalitis, mumps, and embolisms. If he could do those things, then certainly I can hang on through this collapse. He's right. I need to reach in and draw on my will, but it feels so flimsy and flaccid.

I realize, though, in these moments, that I am dying a death of sorts. It's a spiritual death. I sense that this illness, this time of retreat from the world, is forcing me to self-examine, to let go of ways of being and living—even ways of relating—that are not best for me. It was hard to look at this sort of thing when I was so busy living full tilt in the world. I always gobbled up life, did one hundred twelve things in a day, ran two offices, taught classes, wrote my newspaper health column, kept the household in motion, traveled, partied, tended the organic garden, reared the kids, adored my husband. Stepping off the hamster wheel, I see how hastily I lived my life. And I loved it!

This illness is asking a lot of me. It's asking me to change so much of my template. It feels right now like all it wants me to do is give up, give over my varied ways of living my life, knowing myself, sharing with others. I'm at the very edge of my self. Something essential to my soul feels like it's starting to separate from me, like I'm moving away from my own body.

Lying on the green floral sofa, its back against my home's north wall, I gaze across the cherry floors to the low-slung windows wreathed in summer sunshine. My misery is overwhelming. I feel my spirit—or is it myself?—start to lift from my body. I close my eyes and sense I'm taking flight of sorts. I'm leaving. Where am I going? Is this death? But my heart is still beating.

With my eyes closed, my forehead is filling with a picture. It's as if a vivid movie is running in my head. I watch it with great intent. I feel myself floating over the house, looking down on the roof, then inside, glimpsing my weakened form lying listless on the couch, long brown hair draped down my back. I have feelings of sympathy and tenderness for my self, so wretchedly ill. With that I turn my vision north, up the road we live on. I'm gazing above the tall, leafy oaks and bristling white pines toward the string of power lines that lie ahead. With that, I be-come aware that I'm flying, hovering over the trees and heading along the power lines, over the granite rock outcroppings toward the bluing sky and the hills of the neighboring township of Whitewood. *Oh, my God, I'm flying.* My spirit has taken flight. With that, I have a profound aware-ness that I'm not alone. To my right, just off my shoulder, is a grand and stately bald eagle, his snowcapped head beaming in the sunlight. His broad brown wings stretch wide, beating with great strength and grace.

I'm filled with awe as I feel this powerful bird so close to me. As if in a dance, the eagle dips to its left, slipping right under me. The next thing I know we're flying together in tandem, me lying on his shoulders and back, my arms outstretched along his wings.

In some nonverbal way the eagle communicates to me. Words, sentences, feelings arise in my consciousness as if uttered by the glorious creature. I listen internally with rapt attention.

"I'm your ally, Kim. We will fly together now and forever. Trust in my strength and my guidance. I will not let you down. But, in turn, you must trust in yourself, in your own wisdom and intuition, for they're very powerful. This time in your life has been a trial, a test of your inner strength. You have shown great courage and determination in a time of great darkness. You are learning to master the trickery of the mind, the demons that prey on one's soul, the trappings of emotions. I will be with you now, Kim. You have earned your rights of vision. You have been given the gift of eagle's wings. Come soar with me. We will touch the lives of others. Open yourself to the doorway of the divine. You are on the cusp of new understandings. I will be your guide."

I don't know what to think. It seems so fantastical and natural at the same time. My life is so ransacked, with not much else left to lose. I nod yes to the eagle, surrendering to his knowing.

Riding high in the summer sky, we fly over my favorite sequestered pond, deep in the uninhabited woods. I see the sunshine dancing on the crystal water, the leaves shimmying in the warm breeze. My heart fills as we crest the ridge of Lake Pomequit and circle Beaver Pond where Joel and I camped with the children, swimming so joyfully at Old Yeller.

I spy a twiggy nest resting in the topmost limbs of a towering tree. I notice a young, mottled eagle resting inside, its eyes blinking as our sweeping shadow skims by. I sense that this is the nest and baby of my newfound eagle ally. It's all stunningly beautiful, pixel perfect, and anointed with a spell of divinity and magic. In these moments of unheralded vision, I am spellbound.

Eventually, we circle to the west and south, flying for my own home, passing over familiar farms and schools, valleys and back roads. I manage to pick out all of the other residences in which I have dwelled during my time up here in New Hampshire. It's like a summation of fourteen years. The eagle drops down close to the pine tops of the woods behind my home. As we approach my pinprick of a yard, my eagle is gone just as suddenly as he appeared, in a rapid wingbeat of surprise. I hastily descend back into my body lying on the sofa.

"Home, I'm home," I say, stunned and wildly curious about what has just happened to me.

I feel a quiet peace and a strange sense of contentedness. It's as if on my journey with the eagle, I've gained an awareness that if I can stay attuned to my higher power, to divinity, to what people know as God, and not be trapped in the morass of my emotions, I'll find my way out of this snarl of illness. Direction will come to me, answers will be found.

A Gift

The sensations and the eagle's presence felt so real, so tangible, yet I'm not quite sure how to assimilate the experience. I lie still and slightly stunned for a while, finally dozing off for a catnap amid the air-conditioner drone.

Upon awakening I begin to analyze my medical status. In all honesty, I'm seriously ill. Even though the doctors and tests can't ascertain anything beyond an Epstein-Barr outbreak, I intuitively know that something is gravely wrong with me. The nervous system symptoms I exhibit are alarming. The migraines are crippling and, at this point, occur almost daily. In spite of all my nutritional supplements, homeopathy, and acupuncture, I'm not improving in a substantial way. I'm weak beyond words. My emotional state is very shaky. Hunter has used the word "critical" on the phone to my family. Sadly, no one has a clear solution for me.

Something has got to give, I think. As patient as I've been, I feel I need to take the bull by the horns. Even my esteemed homeopathic colleague can't quite find the curative remedy for me. A sudden notion flits through my head. The Indian homeopaths are some of the most skilled in the world. I recall a textbook on clinical homeopathy in my own collection, written by a well-known Indian homeopath, which contains a good section about neurological conditions and effective remedies for convulsions, palsy, and paralysis. It may be of help to me. The problem is that the book is on a shelf way upstairs in the studio space above the garage. Lying here on the couch, this fifty-foot trek feels like climbing Everest. I'm home alone. No one else is around to retrieve the book. I must get it.

I stand up, the room spinning, and inch toward the door. My mind is totally focused on getting up to that bookcase. Wobbly and dizzy, Lucky on my heels, I maneuver over to the garage, propping myself on tables and chairs as I inch along. Looking up the stairs and feeling the oppressively humid heat bearing down on me from above, I consider turning back but will myself forward.

Mind over matter, I tell myself. On all fours, I crawl up the stairs, open-mouthed and panting by the time I reach the top. I haven't seen my studio in over a month. Half-finished canvases call to me. I must ignore them. There's the bookcase off to my right. I crawl over on hands and knees, woozy, heart palpitating.

Amid forty or fifty titles, I scan for the light-blue jacket of *Clinical Homeopathy*, by Anson Jayasuriya, and find it on the bottom shelf. I haven't read it in several years, but I sense that I need its wisdom now. I reach for the book, hands trembling, and take it onto my lap. Upon opening the cover I'm hit with a keen knowing.

There on the blank lead page is an inscription to me in ballpoint ink from an old friend and former colleague, a talented and respected clinical nutritionist who has a great love for homeopathy. For years we counseled one another on difficult cases, subtle gleanings, and remedy differentials. I read his words, now years old:

March 1990. Dear Kim, Best belated Birthday Wishes for Happiness, Success, Blue Skies, and Peace! From one Homeopath to another. I hope this book finds a special place in your life! Best Wishes, Scott.

My heart lurches and I am flooded with a dawning relief. This man is the one I turned to time and again in the past when a case of mine hit a brick wall. With twenty years in practice, Scott's known for his fine intelligence and great gift of helping very difficult cases. I haven't spoken with him in at least five years now.

Scott, I've got to see Scott. He'll definitely know what to do with me!

I tuck the book under my arm, crawl back to the stairs, and lumber back to the sofa. Perusing the neurological section I find two or three remedies that could be of help, matching my symptoms quite closely. The book becomes my new lifeline. Then I pick up the phone to dial Scott's office, his number still embedded in my memory. I'm in luck; his waiting list is often several months long, but as fate would again show its presence, his secretary announces a brand-new cancellation for two weeks from now.

"I just got the cancellation today," the pleasant voice on the phone says.

"I'll take it," I say.

"It's a miracle he's got a space so soon," I tell Hunter when he gets home that evening. I cling to the possibility that help may not be too far away.

Discoveries

I teeter under the weight of the humid, south Atlantic summer blown north. The journey from my front door to the car has never felt so long. Hunter steers me by the elbow, guiding me along our walkway and, at last, into the front seat, where I rest in a fully reclined position for the entire sixty-minute ride to Dr. Scott Worthington's office. Just breathing feels like hard work and that damn shrill buzzing sound is still in my head.

When we finally arrive, the nutritionist's office is cheerful and clean, bathed in soothing sea-foam green and white. Unlike the fluorescent glare of many waiting rooms before this, the lighting here is soft and inviting. There is even an enormous philodendron, which stretches its broad green leaves wide in welcome.

Scott and I are delighted to see each other after so many years, even under such dismal circumstances. I'm very sick and scared, but already sense that I have come to the right place.

"I can tell you the exact day this whole thing started," I begin. "June 21, 2000. My life and health have deteriorated ever since."

Scott asks what happened and I launch into the entire drama. He is all eyes and ears, asking me a few specific questions along the way. "How does temperature affect you? When did the numbing palsy-like symptoms start? Are you retaining fluids?"

After about twenty-five minutes of case intake, Scott makes a confident pronouncement: "I believe this is an advanced case of Lyme disease that has never been treated."

"What?" I stammer. "It can't be. I've been tested three times and all the results have come back negative."

"Did they run the Western blot Lyme test?" he asks.

"They did," I tell him, "all three times."

He nods his head. "But did they run it in the summer of 2000?"

I tell him no, that no one suspected Lyme back then.

Scott shakes his head and lets out a measured breath of obvious disappointment.

"Did they use a local lab?" he asks.

I tell him that I believe they did.

"The commercial lab Western blot is an inaccurate test," he explains, "particularly in old cases of Lyme disease. It's even sketchy in new cases, with a 54 percent error rate. There's a window of opportunity for just a few months when you can get fairly accurate findings with it, but even then, many early cases are missed, too. We need to run some newer, improved tests." He goes on to tell me that some of these are not yet FDA approved, while others are. The good news is that the two labs he recommends are both reliable, state-of-the-art testing facilities. The bad news is that insurance doesn't cover them.

I am astonished to learn that they have diagnosed hundreds of missed cases in the past three to four years, cases that have been mistaken for lupus, MS, fibromyalgia, Parkinson's, chronic fatigue, arrhythmia, all sorts of conditions.

"Is it curable at this stage?" I ask, nervous and elated all at once.

Scott believes that it is. "You've had this likely five years, maybe even more, Kim. As miserable as you feel and all that you've lost, believe it or not, you're not as bad off as some cases I've seen that have been cured."

Tears fill my eyes. I trust Scott completely. After all, sixteen years ago the tables had been turned when I was a young homeopath, aflame with ambition and endless energy, while he struggled through his own long recovery from chronic illness. Now he's the picture of health.

"It'll take some time, Kim, probably two years or so. With a deeply restorative nutritional regime and the proper Lyme's prescription, we can beat it. You may never regain 100 percent of your former stamina, but 80 percent is well within the expected range of recovery. The tests will tell us more."

In addition to obtaining a diagnosis, we need to do several metabolic profiles, fatty acid analysis, and adrenal function tests to assess where the damage has been done. I tell Scott that I don't know what to feel. I'm furious that no one tested me years ago, in the beginning, and I am frustrated beyond belief that all those doctors and hospitals never diagnosed the Lyme.

"What's wrong with them?" I ask. "Why aren't they using these newer tests? For God's sake, Lyme is all up and down the East Coast! I kept telling the doctors that I had this sicky feeling inside me," I tell him. "I could feel something in my bloodstream. Really. My neck would be killing me and I swear I could practically feel a microbe in there. And I get these anxiety spells still, where something very real spurs this physical sensation in my lower back and abdomen and races its way upward through my body. It doesn't start from an emotional feeling. It really feels physical to me. Honestly."

"Lyme could be the crux, or one of its co-infections, Kim. We do need to get some accurate testing done to clarify this."

He says that Lyme can do all sorts of things. "It's difficult for the average general practitioner to diagnose because it doesn't follow one clear-cut set of symptoms but, rather, can attack one or several different systems of the body, depending on the case."

I'm listening acutely to what Scott is saying. After all this time of no answers, this now means so much to me.

"Lyme can show up as musculoskeletal pain and inflammation. It can hit the GI tract. It can be neurological and cause Bell's palsy, vertigo, foot drop, or Parkinson's-like symptoms. It can attack the heart and its valves. With some people it doesn't show any physicals and it goes right to the brain and neurological system, creating anxiety, depression, bipolar, or dementia."

"What a mess," I stammer, suddenly aware of how much worse things could have gotten.

Scott goes on describing this slippery, oft-changing illness. He says that many cases are misdiagnosed or undiagnosed altogether. He considers Lyme to be the epidemic of the twenty-first century, akin to the polio outbreaks fifty or sixty years ago.

I take it all in, nodding in concurrence and a bit in shock. I want Hunter to hear all of this.

While Scott goes to collect Hunter from the waiting room, I sit there feeling gutted, not only by my weakness, but also by the weight of it all.

There are specialty tests to be done at a state-of-the-art interpretive nuclear lab, blood work to be drawn for the protein-reactive Lyme test, and several other tests to request of my general practitioner. We leave Scott's office with a binder of paperwork. I am several hundred dollars poorer than when we arrived, but so much more emotionally filled than I had expected. We've got a direction to explore, some evidence to work with, and, most specifically, hanging in the air like a dancing helium balloon, a potential diagnosis. There is hope.

Answers

D. Pennell is on board with the alternative lab testing, as well as the other tests Scott requested. As he draws my blood, I watch the deep, viscous maroon slowly fill the small glass vial.

How many zillions of prior tests have I been subjected to? I wonder. I pray that this one holds the answer.

Into the protective Styrofoam container the vial goes, padded with ice packs and my paperwork. While I collapse in the car as usual, Hunter overnights the package to a research lab in Florida. A week later, we journey back to Scott's office, and he delivers the results.

"The markers show you are at the very top of the positive range," he says. "You have a full-blown case of Lyme disease. I've never seen a more definitive result."

My heart is pounding in my chest and I feel a sweat break out on the back of my neck. There it is in black and white: 1:128, at the far right end of the spectrum scale. The numbers don't go any higher than mine. Scott explains that I'm infected by the organism called *Borrelia burgdorferi*, the primary culprit in Lyme disease. Somehow, miraculously, I don't have any of the additional co-infections that can be caused by other tick-borne organisms.

I'm crying, clutching Hunter's hand.

"Oh, my god, Scott! Thank you truly. Now there can be an end to this nightmare."

"Let's work on getting you well," he says. "We'll tailor-make a protocol to address some of your deficiencies and help detoxify your system as we kill off the Lyme."

It's going to be a long road, but now I know, at last, where to begin. Relief courses down my shoulders, flowing into my chest, arms, hands, and legs. The tension is drawing and draining, my fear collapsing like a matchstick tower. Sitting in Scott's office, I feel the rivulets of tearful relief trickling down my cheeks. I'm unleashed. No more pins-and-needles nights of gripping fear and days of bewildering confusion. No more crying in the dark or hanging on for dear life. There's a pathway out of this morass. I don't care how hard it is or how long it will take to repair my wellness. We have a diagnosis, a direction, and some options. Lyme is curable! My eagle has guided me here. And mixed within this torrent of relief and budding foliage of joy, there's a cauldron of dark and rumbling anger.

How long have I waited for an answer to this misery? How depressed, despairing, broken, and frantic have I been? How many doctors have shrugged me off without an answer or even an insight into my state of profound sickness? How many months have I held on by the skin of my teeth? Why did I have to lose everything in my life I worked so hard to build because no one did the proper testing on me years ago? Why were five years of my life stolen from me? Why did so many people disregard my pleas for help? Why is chronic Lyme disease so overlooked? Why don't doctors know about these specialty tests?

I'm furious. A rage roils within, dark and powerful like the terrific lashing of a violent gale. I make myself pay attention to Scott, though. It's critically important that I listen to what he has to tell me. I must focus on the steps toward healing. I shove the cavalcade of feelings aside for now.

We carefully go over my other laboratory findings. I learn about the damage that has been done to my immune and nervous systems, as well as to my gut. The Lyme has run rampant within me for at least five years, maybe longer. Though homeopathy and acupuncture have buoyed me in constructive ways, the ugly fact is that *Borrelia* is a virulent bacterium that replicates itself in cyclical fashion. Periods of dormancy can occur, during which time symptoms subside; but then periods of outbreak erupt once again. This spirochete organism burrows itself way into the tissues and cells of the body. Most experts consider it to be even stronger and more difficult to eradicate than syphilis, to which it is related.

"It's a nasty bug," Scott says.

That's an understatement!

He goes on to say that my immune system, once so strong and industrious, has been working in overdrive for years.

"Your low white blood cell count shows how tired and ineffective it's becoming. Because your body has worked so diligently for so long to tackle the Lyme, it has little left to ward off other organisms, leaving you susceptible to these repetitive outbreaks of EBV present in your body. The virus just keeps cropping up, like a herpes outbreak, because essentially you are chronically run-down by the Lyme."

"Well, that makes sense to me," I say. "I get every cold and tummy thing Eli brings home, too."

He says that we need to focus on thymus and spleen support, as well as on rebuilding good flora in my gut to enhance immune response. From there we go on to discuss the extreme magnesium and vitamin D and B complex deficiencies I indicate, as well as my need for essential fatty acids, which will help nourish the nervous system and my very frayed nerves.

"We'll take this as the first step," Scott says. "I want to support the most pronounced areas of depletion first, while we try to mollify this EBV outbreak. After your next visit in six weeks we'll see how you're doing and go about killing off the Lyme bacteria."

"Do I need to take antibiotics?" I ask. I know that tetracycline is the primary one indicated in Lyme disease, but worry about side effects.

"Well, in all honesty, the antibiotics are not that effective in chronic Lyme disease. There's not a lot of evidence that the recommended twelve to eighteen months of intravenous doxycycline and ancillary antifungals and antimalarials do a better job than the powerful Amazon herb cat's claw, which has excellent natural antibiotic properties for killing off *Borrelia*, especially in older cases where a lot of attention to cystospheres is needed."

A part of me just wants to take the drugs and nuke the damn bacteria as fast as I can. I hate these suckers by now. Even Ms. Holistic me is ready to dump the gentler alternative methods and just go for the kill, quick and simple.

"Won't it be useful to kill off some of the active Lyme bacteria now, though," I ask, "and then do in the rest of it with cat's claw?"

"Well, you could do that," says Scott. "You can talk to your doctor about that. But I would advise you not to omit the cat's claw protocol."

He explains that he uses a product called Samento[1], which is the highest, purest grade of cat's claw available now. Apparently, some lower-grade products are labeled as cat's claw[2] but skimp on the amount of the necessary active ingredient. I know what a stickler Scott is for the best-quality products and feel grateful for his high standard of care.

"Okay, I'll wait, and talk to Dr. Pennell, too," I tell him. "I trust you completely, it's just that I've suffered for so long. This disease has ruined me. I'm eager to get well again."

Scott understands. "It's possible that a round of antibiotics could help you feel better initially," he says, "but most Lyme specialists will want to put you on it for a minimum of six months. You'll need to evaluate the consequences of that, knowing how antibiotics destroy the good bacteria, too—especially since your gut is already pretty ransacked. Rebuilding your flora is critical now. I'd hate to see it exacerbated with even a month of drug induction. Talk to your MD; he'll help you figure that option out. But my recommendation is to strengthen you first. Try the cat's claw for a while, and you can always turn to the antibiotics if you feel the need to at any point in time. Building up your depletions is critical now."

"Okay, okay," I say. "I'm ready! Let's get the ball rolling here."

Hunter asks some pertinent questions. We talk more about arresting the Epstein-Barr virus, about the fine balance of needing lots of rest, no stress, and only gentle walks to promote circulation, liver function, and cellular oxygenation. We discuss good food choices for me, and Scott spends a chunk of time emphasizing the importance of solid, long, quality sleep necessary for my recovery. He wants me sleeping between the hours of 10 p.m. and 6 a.m., in rhythm with the body's natural circadian sleep pattern, when the most deeply restorative REM sleep is achieved.

We spend some time reviewing the concept of chronic fatigue syndrome, the involvement of digestive enzyme production, enzyme therapy, mitochondrial function, and depleted adrenal glands. Then, home

---

1 Pentacyclic oxindole alkaloid, or POA
2 Tetracyclic oxindole alkaloid, or TOA

I go with a bag full of supplements, a list of dos and don'ts, and, most importantly, a charted path out of this morass of illness.

I immediately dial Dr. Pennell's office to leave a message for Malcolm, then call my father and tell him the news. Finally, I send out a deliriously ecstatic bulk email sharing the diagnosis with all my friends. When Eli comes home from camp later that day, I tell him the big news.

"Mommy's going to get well, honey. We found out why I've been so weak and sick for so long. One day I'll be well enough to play outside with you again."

"I knew you'd get well, Mommy." Eli grins, then he squeezes me in a tight hug.

Bolstered by hope, I fall into a sweaty, coma-like nap. In those fleeting moments before I slip entirely into unconsciousness, I swear I hear the thump of a powerful wingbeat and feel the graze of feathers across my cheek.

Trudging On

The last month of summer lugs on, drowning us in oppressive heat and humidity. Physically not much has changed yet for me, other than the new arsenal of herbs and supplements I swallow by the handful several times per day. But emotionally I'm buoyed by the elation of my Lyme diagnosis. I'm lifted by dreams of recovery. Dr. Pennell runs a parallel test at IGeneX Labs in Palo Alto, California, another state-of-the-art Lyme diagnostic facility, to see if we can validate Bowen's initial findings.

I discuss the treatment options with him regarding this entrenched chronic condition. Essentially, it boils down to approximately eighteen months of intravenous antibiotics or two years on cat's claw, plus additional herbs such as Andrographis, Astragalus, and Artemisia. We spend time factoring in my low white blood cell counts and Epstein-Barr virus outbreaks, as well as the severe vitamin D deficiency, which Dr. Pennell notes has been a problem for many of the Lyme patients he has treated. He notes that most all those he has tested show radically low vitamin D levels.

"Is this why I always return to improved health after two weeks on a Florida beach?" I ask.

"It very well could be so," he says. "Vitamin D supports immune function, helping you fight off the bacteria and virus. Using a sunscreen SPF of 8 or lower allows you to absorb the sunshine's vitamin D."

Dr. Pennell is an integrative medicine physician, with a heaven-sent genial personality and caring bedside manner. I appreciate his ability to treat the person, not just the disease. Ultimately, we both agree to start with the cat's claw—and-company regimen and see how far it takes me. Our concern about the antibiotics centers on my poor bowel flora and already strong tendency to get yeast infections. If we blast me with the doxycycline bazooka standard protocol, we could be asking for all sorts of systemic complications.

"Let's give you four months on the herbal route," Malcolm suggests, "and see what kind of results we get. You've always lived such an organic lifestyle and are blessed with a strong constitution. With your devotion to natural medicine, you have the understanding and patience to give it a good chance."

I agree.

"We'll keep checking in every six weeks," he says, "monitoring your progress along with Scott. We can always turn to doxycycline if need be. But we need to address the lifestyle changes...."

I thought I had been living carefully before, but in a matter of moments Malcolm shockingly reduces my shrunken world even further.

"Your nervous system is very taxed," he says. "Your immunity and hormones need strong support. Emotionally, you have experienced way too much trauma, stress, and betrayal between this illness and your divorce. In the old days we would sequester you, medicate you with tranquilizers, and hospitalize you for a rest cure. It's critical, Kim, that you look at these next six to twelve months in a similar light. It's a complete rest cure I want you to follow. Minimal involvement in life."

I nod, a bit dumbfounded.

"No cooking, no entertaining, no TV news, no newspapers, no action movies, no going out, no stimuli, anger, upsets. Peace, beauty, tranquility, joy, light-hearted films, lovely novels are to be the norm."

"What?" I balk. "No TV or news?"

"No. They're filled with tension, drama, and upsetting information. I want your nervous system to relax and heal. Just stay at the level of your eight-year-old son. Disney films, romantic comedies, art books, and peaceful, soothing music are best now."

"But I'm trying to get back to cooking," I argue. "Hunter is already so overworked."

"He has to continue to cook. Look for some friends to help with chores. Believe me, it's essential to rebuild you from the ground up. Otherwise chronic fatigue syndrome looms in your future."

"But I'm a maximum extrovert. It's so hard to be alone. I get so sad and depressed with no socializing."

"I don't want you giving out your energy. You need to build up your resources. A visit from a friend here or there is okay, if it's less than an hour. But no driving, grocery stores, errands, or going out to dinner, Kim. Please!"

"Oh, God! Okay," I agree. I know that some of these things are impossible anyway. Computer work and extended phone calls drain me, and the grocery store may as well be Mount Kilimanjaro. I know he's right; I can't handle very much. "Fragile" is a word I have come to know well.

I fill Hunter in on the grisly picture during the car ride home.

"All I can imagine are those neurasthenic Victorian women clad in lacy, lily-white dresses sprawled on chaise lounges, looking wan and distant. I guess that's me now, albeit a tad less elegant."

But he's not upset by the details at all. He promises that he'll help me and that I'll recover. Cozy dinners and candlelight suit him just fine.

Meanwhile, I can't make any progress with the divorce. Joel is being massively stubborn, not agreeing to any sort of reasonable settlement. The volumes of paper and correspondence, negotiations, depositions, subpoenaed business books weave on endlessly like the long, snaking tributaries of the Mississippi. I can't believe the effort that must go into making him budge. Finally, a few weeks later, in a desperate attempt to reconcile, my attorney arranges a negotiation meeting at her office, both lawyers presiding. I'm still deathly weak.

A friend drives me the sixty minutes to my attorney's office, where I spend four hours reclining on an air mattress while the rest of them dicker back and forth in the conference room. Messages and measly offers are relayed to me. I refuse to be in the same room as Joel and all this high-pressured talk. The stress will totally unravel me. Dr. Pennell is against me going at all.

Ultimately, I will not let go of the equity in my house. I purchased that home after my first divorce, before Joel came along, before it became strapped with two mortgages, and before my savings were gouged when neither of us was working. I'm bedridden and still getting no child support. This is a brutal experience, to say the least. Nothing is resolved, and yet the legal fees mount. I return home deflated.

On another front, good news arrives Labor Day weekend. I have a buyer for the house! They exhibit every specification on my wish list: no other home to sell, financially solid, a mature, stable couple with a sixty-day closing date. It's a cash sale, but the offer is a tad low.

"Take the money and run," my savvy father says.

Unfortunately, it will just have to sit in escrow in the attorney's bank. But selling my house is a big step in the right direction. I'm lightening my load, I tell myself. Moving on!

I accept their offer gladly, as my mental wheels spin, imagining a sparkling little spot for Eli and me to move to in town.

The Confirmation

Since my first encounter with my eagle guide, I've been longing to canoe to the back side of Lake Pomequit. It's a favorite spot anyway, but now I'm particularly drawn by the fact that it's the known residence of a pair of bald eagles. Hunter and I have discussed this wish of mine several times now, but we both realize that I'm too weak to make such a journey. Even if he did all the paddling and loaded the canoe with pillows for me to rest on, the ninety-minute outing in open air and water would be too demanding for my very tenuous energy state.

"But I need to see an eagle," I tell him. "It would mean so much to me."

"I know," he says. "It would be magical. But even if we did go, we couldn't be certain that we'd find one. You know that pair is elusive and it's late in the season. They're not as close to their nest now that the young are active and out flying. It's too much of a trip for you with your health. You're still very delicate. Next summer, I promise you, we'll go look for them."

"Next year, next year," I mutter to myself, lying limp on the chaise in my backyard.

For weeks now I've been gazing up into the skies from my back deck, willing an eagle to fly overhead. I want a sign of recognition from the universe that my eagle vision was not happenstance or a mere hallucination. I'm longing for confirmation that the majestic eagle is an ally of mine, but all I see are hawks. Redtails and peregrine falcons soar overhead fairly regularly now in late summer and early autumn. I hear the shrill, piercing cries as they float on the hillside updrafts. But there's not an eagle in view. Hunter's right. It's an extreme rarity to see one. I try to put the wish aside or, at least, to be patient.

Meanwhile, Hunter and I trek faithfully to Dr. Wu's for acupuncture every other week. She, too, is certain from my pulse point's suggestions that the Lyme disease is what has crippled me. And like Dr. Worthington and Dr. Pennell, she is confident that I will get well.

"Remember, constitution strong in you. Condition weakness, not constitution."

"Are you sure?" I ask.

"Absolutely," she says with a matter-of-fact nod of her head and an encouraging pat on my wrist to confirm her belief. "It take time. You be patient. Rest. Take medicine. One year from now you see. Be better."

I pray that she's right, that they're all right. I drift in a semi-sleep, needles fixed on every limb and quadrant, rerouting my chi force and breaking through the spots of stagnation as Chinese music tinkles from the CD player. I let myself drift in relaxation.

Hunter and I decide to come home the back way today, all country roads. It's a more bucolic drive, twisting past old fallow farms and a pretty stretch of rushing river rapids. Though it's less direct and slower than the open commercial route, I appreciate the beauty of the countryside. Close to home and rounding the bend past an open marshland, a massive, dark form swoops right across our windshield. There in broad daylight, plain and clear, is a gigantic male bald eagle. He makes a sharp left turn, skimming over the treetops, and circles back around overhead. Both of us stare at him and his snow-white mantle.

"It's him," I whisper in awe.

"There's your eagle, honey," Hunter pronounces proudly. "You've been asking for him. Here he is showing off to you. You couldn't go to him, so he came to you."

I nod in slow motion, staring up at the sky and the amazing gift of the eagle's flight. Only a few days ago I was bemoaning not being able to take the canoe outing. As the crow flies it's approximately one mile to the pond where the pair nest. My guess is that it is he. In the core of myself I don't question that the eagle has made himself visible to me.

Hunter slows the car. We follow the stately eagle's flight path overhead. He circles the marshland one complete time. I watch his heavy wingbeats, slow and strong, wing tips draping slightly on the downward stroke. He passes over us once more, this time at a higher altitude, heading back to his nesting area. I watch in silence. Nature has spoken to me. I rest assured that nothing is random.

Woodland Home

In a matter of weeks, I'll have to move out of my house. Beginning to fathom the sorrow of my losses, I wander out to the backyard and feel the caress of morning air. I lie on the grass, staring into the vivid blue sky, watching the late summer leaves of the old birch sway. Closing my eyes, I sense the generous homestead of these years and draw it into my soul. I feel the land, my fractured spirit, and the painful fatigue settled in my cells. How sad that my once limitless energy and personal power have been lost.

Lying here I realize that I have to leave the beautiful woods, this home, and my past. I need a new template on which to refabricate myself. In order to break out of the pain, misery, and despair pattern I'm living with, I need to rewire my conscious and unconscious minds. It is difficult for me to retrofit a new circuitry on an old grid. I need a new beginning.

I'm familiar with this necessitated catapult forward from a former plane to a new one, having done this before. Back then, I just leapt from my perch and flew, fearless and free. This time it is more frightening, as I am leaving behind so much of great value, closing a door on all that I had worked to create in my fourteen years in New Hampshire.

My career has been lost, my marriage and family blown apart. I don't see my children every day of my life anymore. I miss Eli's gentle hand in mine, the innocence in Sarah's voice, and Joel's piano chords filling our hearts with song. The finality of it cannot be more visceral.

Stretched out here on the ground, I mutter my thanks to the mighty trees that banked my days and nights for eleven years. I give my respects to the dew-dropped yard and the fertile soil that cosseted the lush vegetable garden that fed the family for so many seasons. The chickens wander quietly. I will miss their soft clucks and proud songs of egg-laying. The fluty trills of the shy hermit thrushes calling forth from the forest floors at dusk will haunt me forever.

The house sits strong and massive on the knoll. It held so much of my world in this tumultuous decade. Inside these walls I watched a baby take his first steps and turn sounds into words. I taught a delicate girl to share her feelings. Here I held many hands, soothed many wounds. People gathered around our long maple table, food and laughter flowing. I embraced it all with honor. I felt graced. Sadly, too, hearts would break and I would crumble.

Now, I bid this home of oak and cherry, of love and heartache, farewell for good. Rising from the lawn, I stumble through the door, lay my weary soul down on the sofa, and fall into a deep, drowning sleep. I await the opening of the door into my next chapter, as I move away from the sickness and suffering, and out of the woods.

Moving

All through the autumn, friends and hired help pack up and ready my house for the move into town. Aunt Connie even flies in from Florida to assist. Hunter makes endless trips to the recycling center, as remnants of my childhood, my marriage, and my ancestors drift out the door in finality, riding high in the back of the old blue pickup.

With me propped on my sofa, pen and notebook in hand, we color-code and catalogue the hundred-plus boxes of kept possessions. The valuable items are off to professional climate-controlled storage, while boogie boards and beach chairs go to the cinder-block self-storage unit. Only the bare essentials will come with Eli and me to our new residence. Paring down to eight hundred square feet is hard and good at the same time. Simplicity has its merits. Blessedly, Eli is on board about the move, eager to ride his scooter on the downtown sidewalks and be so close to school. An eight-year-old's resilience can be inspiring.

Finally, the day dawns, a damp, raw November morning. The house is skinned down to bare bones, dust bunnies floating in the corners. Woozily walking out the side entrance, I feel the finality here, and the thundering clunk as I lock the door for good. Somehow I survive the endless vertical hours. Bull-strong moving men load everything up in their truck and then, just as deftly, unload it all into the tiny Victorian cottage I'm renting. Icy rain taps on the steeply pitched roof. By 3 p.m. I'm collapsed upstairs on my unmade mattress, boxes stacked to the ceiling, not even a drinking glass in sight. But I'm in! I exhale an enormous sigh of relief. Within minutes I hear the squeal of school bus brakes, the rattle of the antique glass in the front door, and then Eli's footsteps bounding upstairs toward me, his new home, and our new life. He's all smiles, blue eyes flashing in wonder, sunny and optimistic about the newness of this big change. My heart swells with his excitement, though I'm overwhelmed by the foreboding task of unpacking and organizing.

The house itself is charmed. We feel it from the very first day. Its energy is storybook-like. In spite of the fact that we're situated at the traffic light and the crossroads of two major thoroughfares, traveled extensively day and night, a certain calm exists within the interior. Our wraparound gingerbread-trimmed front porch offers a sense of protection from the elements and the street scene, while the generous floor-length, lead-glass mullioned windows stream with delightful swatches of golden sunshine. They're so low that short-legged Lucky can peer happily out at the world with ease.

Two small, square living rooms, a newly renovated kitchen, and an airy foyer boasting a lovely old banister railing comprise the downstairs. The ceilings stretch up to a soaring nine feet, from which I immediately hang a beaded violet crystal chandelier, adding further enchantment to the environs. Up the steep stairway sit our two cheerfully sunny bedrooms and a marvelous old-fashioned bathroom, cast-iron tub, etched mirror, and all. It's not a lot, but just enough. Eli and I love this vintage dwelling and take to it immediately. I declare it my "healing house."

Again, friends come to assist me, unpacking, sorting, and alphabetizing the spices. Before long, all is situated. Every nook and cranny of this whimsical house is utilized. We squeeze in bookshelves and space-savers, making the best of what little room we have. With no basement, attic, or garage to pick up the excess, ingenuity is a necessity here. Soon enough, we feel like it's a home we can enjoy. In many ways this small but convenient space is a relief to me.

My energy is still rock bottom. The first hour of awakening is spent readying Eli for school, preparing breakfast, brushing teeth, and collecting belongings. At 8:15 we sit side by side on the staircase, eyes cast out the window, alert for the yellow school bus. As we see its nose poking around the bend, Eli is up like a shot, a hug good-bye at the door, and off he scampers on his way to school. I wave in greeting to the genial driver as Eli mounts the bus steps, then I nosedive onto the sofa. All my energy is drained.

There I float for the next few hours, focusing inwardly on positive thoughts and imagery of my body purging the colonies of Lyme bacteria. I light a candle, put on some soothing music, and stare outdoors at the busy world in motion. Cars and trucks endlessly stream by and walkers take their daily jaunts. I come to recognize various faces and baby strollers after a while, and the timing of certain individual routines. At 10 a.m. a petite brunette passes on her daily run. Close to noon a friend and her two toddlers roll by in a tandem candy-colored stroller. By 3 p.m. our elderly neighbor totes a youngster, yodeling nursery rhymes to the high heavens.

When it's not blustery or frigidly cold, I bundle up and sit on the south-facing porch, soaking in the tepid rays of the midday winter sun. Any bit of sunshine feels like salve to my soul. The sun crosses so low in the sky at this latitude that by 1:30 p.m. it's already ducked behind the roof next door, casting cool blue shadows across my tiny yard. Winter's light is so scarce. I gauge this marking point to be my nap time. Down I go for the next two hours.

I must say that it all becomes comforting to me, living small and within the parameters of this new space. I begin to feel less strained. It's a huge benefit to have Eli riding the bus. My landlords are maintaining the property and snow removal, and the grocery store is within sight of my front door. Everything's in walking distance: the post office, bank, video store, restaurants, though I myself am not walking any farther than my kitchen yet. Having been bedridden for a solid year and isolated in the woods, it is a comfort to have so many conveniences now so close at hand.

Friends often stop in for a hello, colors and sounds enliven me, and soon I'm smiling again. My landlords are two warm and caring foster brothers to me, keeping a watchful eye on our welfare. I feel life and support around me now. Hunter doesn't have to juggle all of it on his own. Sarah still comes over on Mondays after school, the bus dropping her right out front. I'm proud of both of us for keeping our connection intact. With her long honey-brown hair swinging in the shadowy twilight, Eli and I joyfully serenade Sarah on her sixteenth birthday, a yellow-frosted cake flickering with candles. Her endearing smile sweeps love into my soul. What a roller coaster this life is!

Near Christmastime, Eli, Hunter, and I venture out to buy a tree. This is a first for us, as I've always cut a Charlie Brown hemlock from our woods in years past, adorning the tender fingerlike limbs with the Delancey Street market, Hungarian ornaments of my childhood. Now, we mount a generously stout fir, its needles feeling brushlike and full, the wintergreen aroma filling our dollhouse in minutes. Hunter strings up colored lights, weaving the mass through the fragrant branches as Bing Crosby croons carols on the stereo. As woozy as I still feel, my energy dipping and rising with no rhyme or reason throughout the days, I feel a warmth of gratitude within.

After a very long struggle I sense that I'm making progress in my healing. Three months on cat's claw and I'm climbing up from the worst of its clutches. Small signs of improvement bolster my hope: a clearer mind, less stomach upset, and a faint glow of strength in my limbs. The tune from *The Wizard of Oz* has been tumbling through my mind for weeks now: "I'm out of the woods, I'm out of the woods, I'm out of the woods...."

Santa arrives, leaving a slew of boxes. Eli's eyes are star filled as he rips off the vibrant paper, new board games and ice hockey sticks cluttering the room. The quarters are so close we have the Christmas tree placed on top of the coffee table and pushed up against the wall. Teaspoon-sized snowflakes drift down outside the windows. Lucky is festively attired, coyly wearing a brown-velvet antler headband.

"Mommy, Mommy, get the camera!" Eli chants. "Take a picture of Lucky and me."

I capture the moment of perfection.

Sarah stops in for a visit around midmorning, her mom and her mom's longtime beau with her. Like many modern-day melded families, twelve years and dozens of school functions later, Lana and I share a decent friendship. Tea and holiday chatter orbit the room. Blue arrives for gift opening on the heels of their departure. Santa has left gifts here for her, too.

We close the day with a banquet of food, family, and chatter at Hunter's sister's home up the hill. Children, grandparents, and adults with cocktails in hand gather around the burgeoning oak dining table, our number swelling to over twenty. There are smiles and warmth, the feeling of generous embrace from a clan other than my own. There is love.

The tsunami of my life took from me all that was dear, but as the storm waters recede, I see and feel how fortunate we are to have some footing to build on. As we usher in 2006 I peer toward the future. Today, I take my first steps into tomorrow. I reach way deep down inside into the core of my being. From the pit of my belly I draw forth my formerly sagging will. Making a personal pact of intention, I close my eyes and see myself standing upright and strong like a broad-reaching copper beech tree. I'm smiling and radiant. I look and feel healthy and strong, confident and happy, successful and powerful.

I will heal completely, I tell myself. *I will beat the Lyme disease. I will regain my health, strength, and stamina and be whole, happy, and successful. Starting now I leave the past behind and step into a new and joyful future. I will be guarded and protected.*

From today forward I begin to recite my pact of intention each day in my morning meditation, at first prone on the sofa, then sitting, and eventually standing. I refuse to slip back into the downward spiral of all the cataclysmic tailspins over the past five grueling years. I'm determined to heal. No one will stop me. It will be.

Daily Steps

A clear notion has surfaced within me: it's vitally important that I begin to walk again. Though I have kept up a fairly regular
effort of doing some yoga asanas almost daily, even if for a mere ten
minutes, I've barely moved my body during the last sixteen months. Dr.
Pennell finally gives me the okay.

Scarfed in woolens and hooded in fleece, I stumble out the back
door, leaning on Hunter's sturdy arm for support. I manage about
twenty-five steps around the side of the house and in through the front
door. That's it. Back on the sofa to recover for hours. We perform this
ritual daily, managing an extra two to three steps each time. As weak as
I feel, as bitter as the bite in the air, I'm determined. Ten days later we
circumnavigate the perimeter of the yard, about three hundred feet.
Eventually, I make it one block down the sidewalk and back. Later I
increase the journey to two blocks. Finally, we make it to the police station, through their circular driveway, and back into the house, about a
quarter of a mile total. Lucky has now joined me on these outings. I'm
elated and encouraged.

There is finally progress of another kind as well. Joel and I finally
settle on divorce terms with the help of a legal arbitrator. I mentally let
go of my second marriage and treasured family. Twelve years of my life
goes into the file cabinet labeled "history." So much emotion and energy

was invested on many levels. It's a struggle to grasp the death of it all. Now, all I can do is pick up the pieces. I don't know whether to cry or to celebrate. Emotionally, I am bone-tired.

Living on a shoestring with no income makes me terribly insecure. Still, I must not crumble. There is a very dear boy to raise. I hear my mother's words again and again in the wavering moments before sleep, "Stay strong, Kim, and believe in yourself, no matter what."

I force myself to take the daily steps forward, as labored and pedantic as they often feel. I dare not waffle in defeat too long, it is bad for my psyche. The snowfall is light this winter, but the cold is still frigid. Lucky and I continue to walk at noontime, when the mercury makes its greatest ascent. One day, just shortly after my forty-eighth birthday, we actually achieve a mile round-trip. The sloshing clumps of snow spray on us from passing motorists as Lucky and I maneuver around crusty snowbanks and across the slick icy patches. Reentering the warmth of our dwelling, I breathe a wondrous sigh of astonishment at this small feat. I've conquered a mile! Bending to unclip Lucky's leash, he leaps up, his four-inch legs surprisingly springlike, and plants a big wet lick smack on my kisser. I laugh in jubilation, realizing it was three and a half years ago that I bent to hug Echo when she and I finally summited our mountain peak. This small endeavor, in some ways, now feels just as significant to me. Lucky's spontaneity is delightful.

I don't give up the walking. We continue onward, discovering side streets and even hills behind our house. As springtime buds perch sweetly on limbs, fragrant wafts of tulips and hyacinths perfume our walks. Before long, Lucky and I are trudging up and down the spate of hilly streets crisscrossing the western side of town. At spring's peak I realize that my own intention has manifested: I'm walking myself into health!

I actually attend Eli's championship Little League baseball game and watch my feather-thin son pitch the winning final innings in the umber cast of twilight. After a spine-chilling game of epic childhood passage, I startle myself, leaping from my sideline blanket like the Kim of years past, in a whooping cheer, as our victorious team swarms the pitcher's mound. With thunderclaps ricocheting off the surrounding pine-clad hilltops, I hold up during the awards ceremony, but Hunter and a friend must hitch me up by the armpits and limp me back to the car. Nevertheless, I am ecstatic to have greeted the world again.

In the next few weeks the world unfurls into ripe beauty. Now that I have some of my strength back, I desperately yearn to be ensconced on a hillside, stroking tree limbs and cloudscapes onto a canvas. On more than one recent occasion I've even cracked open the top of a tube of oil paint just to look at the rich color and smell the familiar vapors. It doesn't quell the craving, but it certainly stirs the sleeping artist within.

Without warning of any sort, on an especially fine, clear June morning, I get Eli off to school as usual. Hunter is off to a full day of work appointments, not due back until dinnertime. An impulsive rush of energy and fresh enthusiasm race through me. I move quickly through the tiny kitchen, gathering an apple, some drinking water, and a PB&J sandwich. My lightweight aluminum easel and paint bag are in the hall closet. I tuck them into the Jeep, along with a new canvas, a folding chair, and my rugged fedora, and sneak off to a lovely old farm site.

Erecting the easel, I soak in the resplendent beauty of this place. I am filling up with the early summer sunshine, the colors, the smells. As always, I savor the precious minutes leading up to my first brushstrokes. There's something about a blank canvas, freshly mixed paints, and the potential of a creation on my fingertips. This is my favorite moment of plein-air painting. Perhaps it is the excitement, the potential, the discovery that moves me so.

Fifteen minutes into my painting, though, things go awry. My legs are quivering as I stand. My arms are not used to this outstretched position. Soon my shoulders are aching. Ten minutes later I feel a serious fatigue enveloping me. Every muscle hurts and my brain feels waterlogged. I cannot even focus. A moment later I am lying down on the padded cushion of pine needles under a looming white pine. I am too weak to paint. It is a disaster. My spirits drop like a sinking anchor. Tears follow. My beloved artistry as a painter cannot be accessed. It is a crushing blow to find I can no longer even paint. Misery sets in.

Finally, after a spell of despair and sadness, I inch along, packing up the Jeep. On the drive back to my tiny Victorian hermitage, I suddenly recognize the crackling hiss of anger slashing through me like heat lightning. For the first time I feel the voluminous, pent-up rage I've been carrying.

I realize that this anger is very old, gnarled, and seasoned like the rough bark of an arthritic apple tree. I'd known that illness has made me rueful, but until now I have been unaware of just how much I have held within. I'm indignant that I've been stripped of my beloved homeopathy, my artistic work, and my income. It's frightening and humiliating to see the bills mounting around me like billowing circus tents on the open prairie. My medical expenses are astronomical. Migraine medicine is $20 per pill, and I need six to eight each month—along with another few hundred dollars' worth of herbal and nutritive supplements. Doctors, labs, and practitioners are even more. My credit cards are almost maxed out and I'm living on an income below the poverty line, so low that my son qualifies for free lunches at school.

Last week, I bawled hysterically on the phone, sobbing to a laboratory tech when they charged me $920 for testing that my paltry insurance would not cover.

"How can I pay this?" I wailed. "I have no income, only $734 a month from disability. I can't pay this. Help me!"

"We put it on your credit card already, ma'am. You did sign the consent form to bill your credit card. I see your signature here on the paperwork in blue ink," said the neutral voice at the other end of the line.

"But I thought it was less than $300 for the test, not over $900." My heart was shaking, dangling on a thread in my weak, worn chest cavity.

"I'm sorry, ma'am," she said, not sounding very sorry at all. "Maybe you should speak to your doctor."

I slammed the phone down in complete disbelief and frustration, with nowhere to turn.

Now, I thrash the pillows on the sofa, first with my furious outstretched arms, fists clenched, pounding and yelling. My wrists hurt, so I grab Eli's baseball bat. Knees bent, back curled, I repeatedly whack the sofa pillows in a blood-boiling frenzy. Within minutes I'm spent, flopping on the sofa, sobs convulsing my body in a now weary trance. I'm trapped alone within myself in my tiny quarters and the even more constrained relegation to a malingering weak body. It's bizarre to feel so pent up in your own body. No one can bail me out of this mess. I want to give up. It all feels so dire.

I realize that I'm tired of being tired. I'm sick of being sick. I feel finished with all the resting, napping, yoga, gentle walks, and positive imagery! How good do I have to be at all this stuff before I'm granted my freedom from this suffering? I've lost years of my life to this illness.

The dependency is wearing me out and the waiting is torture. I have no more time for this illness. I want to be well and vibrant and active again! I want to paint and socialize and use my muscles, but to run or dance or simply skip feels like a sheer impossibility. I am fuming over all the loss. It's just so much!

I do not know what to do. Stock-still and emotionally emptied, I gaze out from my house at the magnificence and beauty surrounding me. The early flush of summer bathes the neighborhood in vibrant hues, pastel blossoms sweetening the air with their aromatic bouquet. The world around me buzzes and throbs, mating dances in motion, bees at work in the nectar. My thoughts gather in a cumulus column. I try to focus on the positive.

There's natural beauty everywhere I look. Good fortune has brought me a man who loves and cares for me. I have a brilliant son to love and guide. I stare in vacancy into the air, and instantly feel a knowing impulse move through me. Remember the eagle, I think. Listen within. Surely the eagle will guide me.

My eyes are swollen from crying, my throat raspy from sobbing. I move out to the front stoop, where the sunshine bathes me in warmth, and take it all in: the emerald green grass, the stretching blue sky, the melodious birdsong, the glinting flash of sunlight on the cars streaming by. It's life. It surrounds me. It's happening.

I take a dry gulp of air and exhale a heavy sigh. I've come too far to give up. I try to steady my thoughts and calm my palpitating heart. If I don't release this anger, it will eat swiss cheese—type holes in me, setting off depression or further illness. I mentally stuff the ugly feelings into a weather balloon and push it all off into the universe, far away from my mind and body and heart.

There it goes. With my eyes closed, I watch the weather balloon drift, up into the Milky Way. An inner knowing rushes through me: *Keep on trying, Kim!*

Child's Play

"**Y**ou can go down to the pond," Dr. Pennell tells me, "but only floating and dipping are permissible. I don't want you to venture out to the raft, either, Kim. You could still easily overdo it by swimming. I want you on a minimal amount of activity."

I understand, but feel deflated. Will he ever loosen the reins? The summer heat is at its peak and I am eager for some relief. So, every few days we go to the pond, Hunter steadily guiding me down the pebble pathway. Eli dives and splashes with a flock of children while I float on my lime-green noodle and gaze up into the treetops. *At least I'm in the water this year.*

There's something new for Sarah this year: her first boyfriend! Thomas is a fun-loving redhead. The two of them help me out quite a bit, running errands, grocery shopping, and toting Eli to the ball field or off to a fun-filled day at the seaside water park. Blue we don't see quite so much, however, as she is closely cemented to her best friend and busy life at her mom's house. Frighteningly so, the brain tumor is once again showing signs of "activity."

And if the exertion of swimming isn't allowed for me, at least our life in town offers plenty of distractions during these months of prolonged convalescence. Each season here I find a small piece of history or beauty to pique my interest and whet my sense of wonderment. In the spring, tumbling honeysuckle, masses of purple violets, and fifteen-foot-tall lilac bushes bloomed in fragrant echos of a simpler time; I opened all the windows, drowning myself in the perfumed vapors, and adorned each room with armfuls of bouquets. Now, in July, the lovely pink rosebush out front is in full flower. I snip two tender blossoms for my bedside table, placing them in an elegant, etched crystal bud vase.

I learn that our old Victorian has a rich and interesting history. Originally a home and carriage house, over the decades this place has been a realty office, a ladies clothing store, a candy shop, and eventually a curio store. Finally, our landlords purchased the place and restored it to a charming residential space. The former garden and cow pen out back are now a dirt parking lot, where Eli plays sandlot baseball with his buddies and whacks pebbles into the hillside with his yellow plastic bat.

The surrounding homes in the neighborhood are also well-loved relics. The place on the corner is a huge, three-storied grandma of a structure, with an endless veranda and jutting gables dressed in fretted trim work. Catty-corner to that is a well-tended nineteenth-century farmhouse. Its enormous, two-story barn is weathered in a rich amber-and-greige patina, with flower boxes and side gardens brimming in colorful strategy. The place reeks of character and New England charm.

If Lucky is not leashed, he often dashes across the street to the farmhouse on a whim. My heart leaps into my mouth each time he slips through the traffic and scampers behind the barn, ignoring my calls. Often barefooted or, for God's sake, in my bathrobe, I must tromp out to retrieve him. Usually, Don, the friendly neighbor, chuckles, handing the captured pooch back over to me. "Cute fella," he says, giving a ruffle to his fox-thick fur as Lucky pants with corgi mirth.

But Don isn't out front to snag Lucky as he bolts across the street today. Both cars are gone and it is clear that no one is home. Feeling nervous about venturing into their private space uninvited, I wander around to the back of the barn, calling for Lucky, who is nowhere in sight. My flip-flops patter against the bare earth as I venture past high hollyhocks and crimson geraniums.

"Lucky. Lucky," I call.

There is no sign or sound of him.

"Lucky. Lucky!"

Not a wiggle or a peep.

I round the side of the barn, heading down an incline, and catch my breath in surprise. There, smack-dab in the middle of downtown, is a hidden glade. I feel myself fall backward in time and understand why Lucky has taken to running over here at every chance.

The back side of the two-story barn has an open lower level. The thermometer read 90° even before noontime today, but the darkened interior of the barn looks cool and welcoming. I glance to my left and spy an antique leather-top cabriolet-style carriage, its brass landaus and handles dulled with the year's passage. Next to it is a weathered and lopsided wooden cart, its two long pole hitches lying on the ground. I move closer in, thinking that Lucky must have rummaged his way inside here looking for food or critters. But there are no signs of him.

Heading farther into their backyard I am immediately impressed by the enormous spread of the elephant-thick branches on several grand, old sugar maples. They must be two hundred years old. Most of the yard is cooled and shaded by these passive garden giants, even as sunlight plays in dappled splashes beneath their copious awning. The grass beneath my feet is thick and Irish green, the perfect blanket on which to stretch out for a lazy summer nap. I resist the urge.

"Lucky! Come!" I call.

Still nothing.

A few steps farther I find a very pretty stone patio and kitchen garden with rows of herbs, clumps of bachelor buttons, and zinnias, all situated comfortably alongside the ell between the main house and barn, along with bright-orange tiger lilies and sweetly scented ferns as a backdrop. Where the lawn meets the patio there sits a large, old-fashioned washtub filled with clear, glistening water and a prim clothesline dotted with freshly laundered shirts. It's like a walk back in time.

The yard is surrounded by a shoulder-high barrier of witch hazel and viburnum bushes, abutting the river, which ambles amiably through town on this stretch. I marvel that this one-acre plot can feel so peaceful while traffic buzzes by just a stone's throw away. *Lucky must be down by the water,* I think, turning to the direction of the camouflaged river. A rope swing hangs from a sturdy branch of one of the maples, its wooden seat speckled with flecks of sunlight.

I glance about, still seeing no one at home, then alight on the swing as freely as a butterfly, pushing my toes into the warm grass and propelling myself backward. Instinctively, I dip my head and shoulders back, my long hair dangling downward and feet stretching upward to the sky. Gliding forward on the swing, I catch a piece of blue above the treetops. Back and forth I sway, gaining momentum with each pump of my legs. Suddenly, I am a schoolgirl again, absorbed in the freedom of play.

Swinging so freely makes me aware of how cooped up and serious I've become during these years locked in the straitjacket of Lyme disease. *Loosen up, Kim,* I coax myself. *You're becoming so tamed and tempered. Enjoy yourself!* But, it's so hard to feel breezy when you've been so sick, forever. Soon I remember that I am here to fetch Lucky. Dragging my feet, I slow to a stop.

I search for a break in the bushes where a dog may have ventured toward the river. Seeing a likely spot at a tiny gap in the lower witch hazel branches, I push myself through the greenery and enter into the stubby growth of saplings and the marsh dock of the wetlands. About twenty feet ahead, caked in mud up to his belly, stands my wayward dog, eagerly sniffing the flowing river.

"Lucky, for God's sake, you are so stubborn," I declare. "Bad dog! In the house!" He looks up at me sweetly, simultaneously grinning and panting. I feel the joy he is relishing, escaped from his dominating leash. I exhale deeply. Instead of insisting that he get back to the house as I usually would, I join Lucky at the river's edge, sipping the new medicine of fun. Off come my flip-flops and we wade in together.

Time to smell the roses, I think.

We eventually make our way out of the wetlands. Traipsing across the bucolic glade one last time, we come upon Don, returned home. I relay the story of Lucky's escape, but keep the swinging secret to myself. Don laughs off our episode and Lucky and I head back across the street, where we collapse inside the air-conditioned comfort of home. Just those twenty minutes of exertion have drained me. *Dr. Pennell is right, I still need to pace myself.*

Even with these strides I am making, and the parcels of joy I experience, I am still only half the person I used to be on so many levels. I sense that I need to move forward more with my healing, but how?

The Next Step

Imanage a minor outing about once per week, maybe venturing to the post office or taking a walk to a pretty spot behind the Dunkin' Donuts down by the riverside. I have come to cherish this spot, only several hundred yards from our home, as a vantage point for observing the seasonal cycles. We've watched the water grow more sparse and then the mosquitos thrive in the mounting rains and, now, the arrival of mallard ducks in the shallows. Eli is entranced by this little glimpse of nature, too, skipping stones or coaxing Lucky in to retrieve a ball. Yesterday we found a bush of elderberries picked over by the birds. Still, though, most of my time is spent splayed out on my ship of a sofa, the hollowness still present in my chest.

One day, out of the blue, a letter arrives from the Stillpoint School of Integrative Life Healing. A friendly note is enclosed and includes all the information about the upcoming yearlong training program, as well as some weekend retreats to be led by Meredith Young-Sowers. This is the Meredith from my past, the one I visited years ago for the migraines.

What uncanny timing, I think. An inkling of hope and curiosity sparks in me.

I lie motionless, rereading the letter several times, imagining all that I might learn about intuitive healing if I could go to this school. By now, Meredith has written several more books, produced healing CDs, and more. The magnitude of her healing wisdom has touched thousands around the globe. The lovely blonde woman I sat so serenely with in the garden has spread her wings and flown far and wide, sharing her talent and love.

Trembling, I dial the school and speak with Kit, the program director. We schedule a healing session for me with Meredith, to find counsel on my weakened state of chronic fatigue. A few days later Meredith speaks with me at length on the phone and shares insights about my blocked creative energy and need to "rewire" the focus on my life's work. Her empathic words of advice are like a life preserver to me. I have obviously stuffed my ambition and abilities into submission during these years of collapse.

"Do not worry, dear heart," she kindly encourages. "You are doing some very powerful, internal work there on your sickbed. Your subconscious is trying to connect with your conscious mind, asking you to change. Be patient with yourself. It will come together. The healing exercises we just spoke of will assist this process. Love your self, Kim. This is very important to accept."

Tears brim in my eyes. I so want to be well! Tentatively, I inquire about the school program, my soul still longing to attend.

"We're waiting for you to join us. I know how much you'll gain from the whole experience."

"Oh, I so much want to come," I tell her, "but I'm so weak still. It's just so hard now."

"Things will work out, dear heart," she replies. "Your life is changing rapidly. Hold on to your will to heal."

Her encouragement bolsters my hopes.

Although I'm still at half-mast, in the ensuing weeks I begin to contemplate seriously the idea of attending the Stillpoint program. I'm simultaneously excited and scared about the whole thing. I contact Kit again and she encourages me to submit my application for schooling even though I'm uncertain about my health and the financial means.

"Let's hold the intention that you'll be well enough to attend, Kim. If not, you can always defer to the next year," she suggests.

"Okay," I reply, fingers and toes crossed that I will somehow build up the stamina to manage a five-day residency four times a year at a facility far from my home, without all my routines that help to keep me buoyed. *How can I survive the travel there and back? No daily two-hour naps? And can I sustain all the at-home course work between resident sessions? Plus how can I create a budget schedule to pay for this schooling?* For a disabled person it feels like an enormous undertaking, but my willpower bites down hard on Kit's application suggestion.

"I will go!" I doggedly declare. Hunter supports the idea complete-ly, knowing how broken my spirit has been. We both realize that I need to address the emotional ravages of the illness as much as I have the physical. Until I mend my spirit, I can't be truly well. Healing is not one-dimensional.

And so, I begin to "imagine" myself going to this special school. On and off at varying times, in my mind's eye, I visualize myself sitting in a classroom with Meredith presiding. I conjure images of me walking with oomph in and out of buildings there. I so want to attend! I will a version of this possibility into my consciousness. It becomes a small ritual of mine, actually. I write the word "Stillpoint" on a piece of paper and tape it to the bathroom mirror, saying it out loud each time I glance at it.

A few weeks later, at my scheduled visit to Dr. Worthington, we re-view my status and talk about what approach to pursue next at this level of recovery. I hope he has some supplements that will boost my energy.

"I feel a general trend of improvement," I tell him, "but I'm still dealing with the fatigue and body pains. The ache in my neck and hips can be fierce. Some nights it's so bad that I have to take a pain pill to sleep. Will I ever get back to my old self?"

He assures me that I will eventually get much of my former energy back, but that I will need to shift my expectations and pace.

"I remember telling you twenty years ago that you needed to slow down!" he says. "You used to thrive at a high tempo, Kim, but it wasn't really healthy for you. Most everyone needs to downshift as they ap-proach the age of fifty, and with the long-term ravages of chronic Lyme, I don't see that you'll have a choice. My guesstimate is that you'll be healthy and satisfied at around 75 to 85 percent of what you used to think of as good or normal energy."

That may be his opinion, but I want to believe in a better outcome. "I feel now like I'm moving at a snail's pace," I tell him. "Hunter says that it's an important life lesson I'm learning."

Scott agrees, but assures me that we can manage the pain.

"I'm going to have you try an herbal formula called Kaprex, which contains rosemary and oleanolic acid," he says. "There are no known side effects, and other patients of mine have adored it."

He also gives me a supplement for mitochondrial support, to enhance my energy.

"That sounds good," I say hopefully. "And listen, Scott, I've been wondering about the Rife machine I've heard about. It's supposed to be so helpful with Lyme. I've known about it for years and lately read about its use with other Lyme sufferers. What do you think?"

Dr. Royal Raymond Rife, a scientist-physician at the Scripps Institute, originally created the Rife machine back in the 1920s as part of his work to cure cancer. By using a powerful microscope fifty times more accurate than others of the time, he was able to identify microorganisms never seen previously. This research led to two enormously valuable discoveries. The first is the Rife technology, which involves the use of electromagnetic energy vibrations and patterns to eradicate illness states. The second was his discovery that all cancers originate from a blood virus that breaks down cellular function in such a fashion that the consequences are irregular cell growth in the form of tumors.

The Rife machine's effectiveness was duplicated numerous times in the span of a rigorous decade of research. Dr. Rife's colleagues were overcome by the success of his obvious discoveries. But tragedy followed Rife and his scientific breakthroughs, including the dubious disappearances of his colleagues and the early machines, and the technology all but disappeared into obscurity.

As a result, no money or attention has been designated to understand fully the dynamic workings of this once highly praised technology. We're way behind on the learning curve here in the USA regarding Rife technology, as the FDA has yet to approve its use for medical conditions—hence, the "experimental" status Rife technology is given presently in our country. But I have read that many people swear by its success in obliterating the Lyme bacteria from the body.

"I think it's good stuff," Scott says. "Do you recall Dr. Prescott, the well-known nutritionist from the seacoast?"

"I remember his name."

"Well, he suddenly closed up his practice and vanished one day. It was an unprecipitated disappearance. After about a year or so he showed up, claiming to have retired to California, but apparently he was struggling with a severe case of Lyme disease. He turned to the Rife technology and says it's what cured him."

Very interesting, I think. I ask Scott whether he has any idea where I can find a machine.

He says that you can get them in Canada and over the Internet, of course. The FDA hasn't approved them here in the States yet, so it's all considered experimental right now and the machines are very expensive, around $2,000.

"Why don't you ask around?" he says. "I'll do the same. Maybe you'll find one to borrow. Try it first to see what it's like."

Through some searching I'm able to borrow a small and rather unimposing Rife machine. It's a manageable boxlike form, about 6x8x4 in dimension, with a numeric keypad on the top face. Two wire cords extend from plug-in points, with cylindrical stainless steel wands at the ends. It plugs into a regular 110V AC socket. The machine is programmable via the keypad. A companion booklet identifies the energy frequencies available to address hundreds of illnesses and states, including emotional ones, like fear and forgetfulness. Treatment for simple problems such as fatigue, hemorrhoids, premenstrual syndrome, and jet lag is available as well.

I'm very eager to give it a try. Turning the pages I find *Borrelia burgdorferi,* the primary Lyme bacteria, clearly noted in the booklet as frequency code 26. It's recommended to start initially with four minutes two times per day, working up to sixteen minutes per day. Plain and simple. I plug in the Rife machine, grasp the wands, set the machine to #26, and dial the modulator to the lowest level of stimulation so as to see what it feels like. I note nothing. I gently dial the modulator up and experience a buzzing sensation in my hands like champagne bubbles. It's not unpleasant. If I dial it farther up, the electrical stimulation becomes too intense, making me want to drop the wands. I find my point of comfort and wait the four minutes out. During that time I note a subtle up-and-down cadence to the frequency, delineating an energy pattern. For curiosity's sake I try a few other frequencies. I choose the ones for fatigue and migraine, trying to sense any difference between them. Sure enough, each one vibrates in a different manner. I'm intrigued.

Hunter and I spend the next week poring through the manual. There are various recommendations for running additional frequencies such as "body detoxification" and "kidney cleanse" while using this technology, so as to help eliminate the dead bacteria and associated toxins from the system as the offending microorganism is killed off. The booklet also recommends lots of pure water, rest, and good food. Chemical over-load, geopathic stress factors, and impure foods, it says, set up breeding grounds for organisms and illness to thrive in. I realize that embracing the Rife technology is an entire healing system in itself. It's quite a wonder, really. Being a classical homeopath, relying on finely attenuated vibrational remedies for years now, I can accept this concept of energy medicine as something that could be viable.

Within two weeks on the Rife, I notice a truly substantial improvement in my energy. At the one-month mark, it's dramatic. People are commenting on how well I look, how much clearer my eyes are, and how much energy I seem to have. I find it quite striking to experience these changes so much more quickly than I'd expected. Hunter and I are both tickled with this marked advance in my healing.

As the leaves descend from the trees, gathering in dense clumps around the neighborhood, Lucky and I are walking farther and faster than before. The once arduous half-mile trek down to the post office is now an easy saunter. We climb the steepest street in town with ease. I even dare to invite company over for spaghetti dinner for the first time in more than two years. I'm totally impressed by the Rife's effects, but simultaneously I don't dare stop the cat's claw and other supportive supplements.

Snowfall comes early, in late October, dimpling our cement side-walk and layering the vermillion-red burning bushes in a frosted coating. Sadly, though, the on-loan Rife must go back to its owner. In a fury of web searches, phone calls, and hours of online research, I'm able to find a used Rife machine. After pleading with my father and chronicling the stunning success of the Rife's workings, he willingly buys me the used machine as my early Christmas gift. I'm both relieved and elated. In the few weeks since I had to return the loaner, I've noticed a true loss of progress. Now, I sit "plugged in" nightly as we watch benign TV comedies. I still omit the evening news.

It's interesting how being uninformed about the world at large has not been a hindrance in any way. *Less mess, less stress,* I realize. Instead of worrying over world events, I sit calmly, champagne-buzzing sensation in my palms, watching Disney movies with Eli. The din of cars cruising by outside, the smell of baked potatoes wafting in from the kitchen, and the glowing windows of fire-stoked houses in the neighborhood quell me in comforting ways. I feel a warmth, a smile within.

Initiation

In late autumn, Hunter chauffeurs me two hours north through a torrential downpour to the Stillpoint School of Integrative Life Healing. The Rife machine is tucked in with my other necessities: a portable camping air pad, a down pillow, and my sack of vitamins and herbs. The work of the Rife machine has given me the strength to finally take on this experience.

Hunter leaves me at the school's door. After a hug and a kiss and a wave good-bye in the raven-black night, I sense that I'm on the threshold of a whole new dawning. The tall oaks nod secretively to me, the wind whisking the royal-purple scarf from my neck as I slowly ascend the steps of the carriage house. Stepping inside the Stillpoint chambers, I smell the familiar scent of woodsmoke and hear the lilting voices of people gathered. Candles flicker, floral bouquets color the classroom tables, and the cathedral ceiling stretches high, its strong wooden beams glowing in the firelight. This is like no other school I've attended. Its radiant aura envelops me. A warm hand presses mine, and I turn to recognize the eternal beauty and delight of Meredith, her lovely face smiling at me.

"Welcome, Kim. You're here," she proudly says.

"I finally made it!" I declare. "It took me eight years from our first meeting, but I'm really here."

"Yes, you really are here, dear one, I loved your application essay. You're a beautiful writer, Kim."

"Oh, thank you. It's all those years of practice with my health column," I say, brushing off her compliment in my insecurity.

"It'll be a wonderful year for you," she offers.

"I do hope so," I say, soaking in the magical ambience of this charmed carriage house, the crowd of people in attendance, and the imaginings of what lies ahead for me.

Soon, the evening session starts. Standing in a large circle, thirty-five Stillpoint initiates each hold a single white candle. The roaring fire crackles, the electric lights are turned off, and transcendent music fills the room, lifting my heart in a spiral of goodness. A feeling of reverence is growing as Meredith, our doctor of divinity, speaks an invocation of welcome and intention to us. We all rest in silence, soaking in the growing awareness of spiritual presence. A sizable photograph of the spiritual leader Sai Baba rests on the rustic wood fireplace mantel. On the opposite end sits a black-and-white image of Jesus Christ. A few other items, such as a mandala, prayer shawls, Tibetan chimes, and a Buddha statue dot the room. All religious and spiritual belief systems are respected here. But this experience is not about religion; it's about spiritual healing and the development of our intuitive skills. The opening ceremony does not gloss over the understanding that certain powerful spiritual and religious figures possess vast intuitive strengths. We hold their images within our company in recognition.

The evening flows on with Meredith guiding us through the focus of our year ahead. We touch on the conceptual process of the skills we will come to master. Meditation, prayer, movement, creative expression, laughter, and love, silence, and writing will be the important vehicles we will come to rely on. At the evening's end we each stand and state a simple, self-selected word of conviction to embrace on the lip of this journey toward inner healing. I speak the word "strength," my legs quaking under me in a tandem of fatigue and anticipation.

I scan the room, seeing faces of all ages and countenances surrounding me. A bohemian-spirited brunette sparkles in beads and golden jewelry, while a sleek silver fox speaks in a powerful, confident tone. A shy slip of a lamb keeps her eyes downcast, standing next to a proud, square-shouldered man of steady composure. I see wheelchairs and walkers. I have my air pad. There are faces filled with light and hope, others shrouded with dark shadows of pain and leathery sadness.

I'm awash in a kaleidoscope of feelings. My wounds are palpable and fresh, lying millimeters under my skin, too raw for even me to touch. Yet I feel so grateful to have found this remarkable school and the opportunity to explore a new dimension in healing. I'm scared and eager both. Insecure yet sensing I'm doing the right thing, even alone here in the New Hampshire highlands. I feel a beautiful outpouring of love in this room.

As the session closes, Meredith comes and stands in front of each student. She gazes deeply into our eyes, truly seeing the unique beauty within each soul. She lights our individual candles, uttering a few words of blessing, then moves quietly to the next person. Soon the space is basking in the buttery glow of candlelight. I feel anointed.

Spiraling In

While in residence at Stillpoint, we are housed high up on a hillside, dormitory style. My room faces east with a spectral broad-reaching view stretching across an undulating valley, touching on a distant mountain range. As dawn breaks, I watch a pumpkin cast of light rise along the ridgeline, streaming a glowing band of light into the world. The wind whirls a morning breath through the delicate needles of the strong white pines. I sit motionless on the bed, breathing ever so slowly, taking in the purity of clear mountain air and the gift of this priceless new day.

I think it's a wise choice that Meredith has brought us up into the northlands to seek and study. There's little distraction from society and commerce here. We're immersed in tranquility and the endless beauty of nature. A great peace settles within me. But still, I'm anxious as to how my stamina will hold up in the full nine-hour-plus day ahead of me. I check in with my body before dressing. I feel the usual tremulousness and tired weight on my chest. My spirit, however, is so eager to go to class and learn that I override the weakness with my emotions and push myself forward into the day.

Our first agenda is morning meditation. While immersed in it, I feel deep and rooted. After Meredith's inspired morning lecture, we spend a good part of our day exploring a suite of eye-opening exercises, all of great significance. Intuitive training is exciting work. Meredith is helping us to enter into the right hemisphere of our brain, the side of images, sensations, language, and gut hunches. We learn how to hone our perceptions, trust our instincts and reflexes. Much of this work stimulates the pineal gland. This often overlooked endocrine gland sits quietly in the center of our forehead. It has long been associated with spiritual knowledge and what some consider the sixth sense of intuition.

Our day is chock-full. By lunch I'm abuzz with insights, self-discoveries, and a handful of new friends. We've come from all over the globe to study here: New York, Ohio, Indiana, Canada, Paris—the list stretches on and on. People from a broad variety of careers are represented. I marvel at our diversity: computer programmers, nurses, writers, teachers, therapists, dancers, business managers, and artists. Our common thread is an interest in alternative healing, specifically in the dimension of emotional and spiritual work. Many of us are personally in crisis, others are merely curious seekers, and some are veterans of Stillpoint, back to iron out a few wrinkles. What strikes me so vividly is the genuine kindness everyone emits.

It's a pleasure to be in the midst of so many people who are inclined to venture into the often uncharted regions of the self. I sense an immediate chemistry with many of these complete strangers. Our backgrounds are varied, our bodies sometimes struggling, but each and every person I speak with has a bright, clever mind and a brave, sensitive heart. *What a wonderful conglomerate of folks we are,* I think, inching my way down the pathway back to our classroom after lunch.

Periodically, I must lie down on my air pad during the afternoon lectures and exercises. We're in the heart of my daily nap time, yet I dare not miss a venerable word of Meredith's teaching. She inspires and guides each student with a finesse that infuses logic and mystery into tangible results. Our exercises are practical and foundational, drawing on an enormous array of abilities and understandings I have sensed but never knew how to harness.

We learn how to turn to our perceptions, using images as metaphors for understanding and answers. Apparently, many people shy away from their intuitions, out of fear of not belonging, or doubting themselves. Meredith shows us, in a seemingly simple exercise, just how influential symbology and our internal powers of perception and self-awareness really are.

"Please, all of you get comfortable in your chairs," says Meredith in a steady, soothing tone. "Sit with your feet square on the ground, backs straight, arms relaxed. Let's all close our eyes." The room grows still in these silent moments.

"Steady your breathing to a slow and deep rate. Concentrate on bringing your breath way down into your belly, not just up in your chest. Let's do four or five breaths like this...."

We follow suit.

"Let your mind follow your breath as you inhale and exhale. Just put your focus on this now. Relax your muscles. Find an inner quiet. Nice. Now, bring your attention into your chest and touch into your heart. Feel its warmth and presence."

By now I'm mellowed and loose, supple as olive oil. We all breathe quietly in silence, absorbing the directions.

"Place a hand over your heart. Focus your concentration there."

I feel my focus dropping into my chest, tuning in to the bumpity-bumpity rhythm of my heartbeat and the awareness that my heart does occupy a place in my chest and actually seems to glow a bit energetically.

"Give thanks to your deep heart and its knowing," guides our seasoned teacher. "It houses your life force and your love. Feel how important this love is, how valuable this seemingly small yet very industrious organ is, propelling your blood and oxygen throughout your body. Recognize how special the heart space is. It holds our love and is the center of our truth and knowing."

I feel choked up, realizing how much love we store within and how we often skimp on expressing it, both to others and to our very own selves. I see how shuttered my heart has become in recent years. My, how open and generous I once was with my love. I see a flashback of me, running open-armed, smiling wider than the hills, into the outstretched arms of my first husband, his tall boxer's frame engulfing me in a feet-off-the-ground twirling hug of passionate adoration. It shocks me to find he's still stored in my heart space, fifteen years later, considering the violence and danger that ripped us apart. I'm jerked back to the present as I hear the silken words of my teacher.

"Good. Trust yourself and feel the love you bear. We're all going to do this exercise together now. There's no right or wrong way with this. Trust your impressions, responses, feelings, and visions. We'll write them down and discuss them later. Right now I want you just to relax and receive. Don't judge yourself or what comes to you, even if it's a seemingly minor or insignificant image or feeling. This is all a process," she encourages us in her gentle yet matter-of-fact way. "Keep your eyes closed, your breathing slow and steady. Let's stay relaxed and open."

I feel excited and curious about where we're going and what we're doing right now. I'm in a semi-trance, on the verge of falling off into sleep, but not really. It's obvious I've dropped into a deeply restorative theta brain-wave state.

"I want each of you to think of a question you would like an answer to. Nothing too complicated. A simple question, such as 'How can I make more money?' or 'What can I do to improve the communication with my son?' Take a couple of moments and compose a question internally."

My mind wanders for a bit. There are so many topics I want advice about: my health, relationships, money, Eli, my dad, my future. Skimming through this array, I settle on a rather specific question, an idea I've been toying with: "Should I write a book about chronic Lyme disease?"

"Hold your question within for a moment more," she guides us. "Shortly, we will open our eyes. When I instruct you to do so, I want you to notice the first thing your vision falls on. Just take that in and be with it for a minute or two. Notice the object, the colors, any small thing, no matter how seemingly insignificant, that catches your awareness. It may be a flower in the vase on your table, a book in front of you, a piece of the fireplace ahead. It does not matter. Just accept that initial perception and stay with it."

I'm holding my question square in the center of my mind now.

"Gently and slowly, with a soft gaze, open your eyes," Meredith continues her directive.

I gradually lift my heavy eyelids. My gaze falls eight feet or so ahead of me onto the small table next to Meredith's chair. I see a lit red candle.

"Now, take a few minutes and write down some words about the item you alighted on, any feelings and any details that came to you. This is free form and spontaneous. Don't think about it at all. Logic is not our guide here; impressions are."

I write down the following words:

> A single red candlestick, burning with a clear flame. Simple and bright, clear and standing erect. A pink ribbon lies next to it, slightly to the front, bent at an angle. The candle rests in a yellow-gold base. I'm happy it's lit. It looks beautiful and comforting, illuminating, and somewhat sacred in a way.

A few minutes later Meredith continues, "Now that you've described what you saw, let's take some time to sense what any of this symbolism could communicate to you about your question. Again, I don't want you to get too analytical or literal here. Put your hand over your heart again and settle back into your deep heart space of knowing. If it helps to close your eyes, please do. Read your own written words to yourself. Feel anything that arises within you, whether it's a thought, a sensation in your gut, words running through your head, anything will suffice. This is not like a scientific formula or a math equation; it's following our own impressions."

I read my words once to myself. I place my hand over my heart and close my eyes. Immediately, the image of the burning red candle and the angled ribbon reappear. A quick series of thoughts flow through me. I gather them. They feel very solid and right to me, more so than usual.

"Would some of you like to share your experience with the rest of us?" Meredith inquires. "We can all learn from one another. Let's hear some of the questions and discovered images, and the impressions that arose within you. We'll see what kind of information there is to work with. Again, there's no right or wrong."

One woman speaks first. We're all captivated at how her image and the feelings associated with it are a direct route out of a dilemma she faces. I get up the nerve to share my exercise, too. The portable microphone is passed hand to hand along the room to me. I state my question out loud and then speak about my eyes alighting on the lit candle and accompanying ribbon.

"What kind of impressions and interpretations did you collect from this image as relates to your question?" Meredith asks me.

"Well, the first thing that struck me is that I can hold or bear a symbol of light, in my effort to tell my Lyme disease story," I more or less insecurely utter. "Like I can shed some illumination on the subject or the experiences of this difficult illness, since a candle represents light and illumination. If the candle represents me, well, I guess I sense that my book will burn bright and that I can stand tall and proud with it."

"Nice. I like that. What else did you sense? Anything about the colors you noted or the ribbon you mentioned to us?" Meredith extracts.

I feel what surfaces within me. "Ummm. The ribbon is near the base of the candle, which is a yellow-gold square shape. The ribbon is pink and kind of at an angle, and touches a white piece of paper in front of the candle."

"And what about all that is helpful to you, Kim?"

"My feeling is that I must come into the story from an angle and follow that as a way to communicate. Then it will lead me to a position of strength and, ultimately, some sort of light. Oh, I get it!" I burst forth. "I must weave the story together, like a ribbon bends and curls. It shouldn't be just a straightforward, science-based book, but one that follows a path—my path."

"Very nice. How does that feel to you, Kim?"

"Great!" I say as the lightbulbs go off inside me: I do have a rather phenomenal tale to tell, one that could shed light on other people's lives and similar suffering.

"Let's not overlook the colors here, either, Kim. Any reaction or hunches about the red, yellow, pink, and white?" encourages Meredith.

"I don't know that much about color, other than I love colors and my paintings are loaded with vibrant hues. Pink represents love, right? Maybe I need to commence the story from a place of love and beauty. I should start it from a clean slate, like a blank piece of white paper." The words escape from me.

"Yes, that sounds right. Can you think of a starting point in your life, or this story, that was a clean slate and you were surrounded by or living within your love?"

"Completely," I reply. "I'll start it off on the magnificent day I initially got sick, summer solstice 2000. Now I see the message of the blank piece of paper and the ribbon of love. Very cool," I say, shaking my head in wonderment.

"And we must not overlook the fact that the candle is red and sits in a yellow base," Meredith says. "Yellow is the mind and ideas, often ushering in information. My sense is that you do have a great deal of information on which to base your book. Red represents the heart and passions. It's suggesting that your strength and upward movement, or progression, in both the telling of this story and in your own healing, will be best explored by following your heart and communicating with passion. It's that passion that bears the light of illumination. It's your heart that burns bright. From your heart you will heal." She nods and smiles at me in a quiet, respectful way.

I sit motionless and vibrating within. I get the deeply centered feeling that I must begin this writing. It's as if a precious, elegantly wrapped gift was just placed in my outstretched hand. I'm awestruck.

Next, a brilliant realization thunders through me. This tuning in to the self through the deep heart is a wiser way to make a decision. I seesaw over so many things in life, decisions as minor as which dress to wear to a dance, or as enormous as should I marry this particular man or not? Shit! I have been so off balance for decades, I suddenly realize. Who teaches us how to tune in to our knowing hearts in this culture? We've been schooled to rely on our intellectual minds. Religion tells us to have faith, but in a source outside ourselves, not this mighty wellspring within. I'm practically shuddering, suddenly in panic and distress at how I and so many millions of others have been denied the ability to trust our own gut hunches and, worse than that, to not develop these innate skills. Developing them is not hard. This simple little exercise has opened up a window once slammed shut inside of me.

In some ways I'm beginning to see that the "picture stories" my mother shied away from in my childhood are the very sort of matter Meredith is teaching us to garner. It's actually liberating to find out that fleeting images, sensations in one's belly, or a random knowing don't need to be pushed away or disregarded as I did in the past, but should actually be examined and trusted as insightful. I feel a tornado of relief.

We go on in the following days to learn about the body's seven energetic chakra sites and the interplay between emotions and physical illness. I'm struck by the amazing conduit of influence we personally possess within ourselves to promote healing. I've spent twenty years of my life devoted to helping others heal. In many ways I've spent my entire life as a healer, nursing animals in childhood and aiding friends in need.

All my years as a homeopath, listening to and assessing other people's woes, perfected in me the art of compassionate listening. But now, here at Stillpoint, I'm learning that there's so much more to true healing. I'm discovering the incredible riches of the spirit. A profound wellspring is available to those who can find the still point within themselves, their own reservoir of unquenchable healing love. Changing one's conscious thoughts can potentially induce a neurochemical and hormonal cascade that will promote the body's healing response. I am wonderstuck.

The Stillpoint Model of Healing is a stunning piece of work. We begin to practice all its varied techniques on ourselves and one another in working pairs and group sessions. Over and over, throughout the day, I'm overwhelmed. I experience jolts of self-understanding as we work our way through personal issues of pain, confusion, and fear, and I feel my heart opening to genuine grace.

Meredith teaches us how to enter the coveted sanctuary of our deep heart, a space of profound trust, safety, and knowing. Monks, nuns, and mystics across the ages have diligently worked on preserving this sacred space within. It's the space of connection to the divine, the source of inner knowledge. I first learned about this treasured place of inner light during my thirteen years of Quaker schooling, but the knowing got quickly trampled once I entered the hectic life of adulthood. Our frantic, goal-oriented culture drives us away from our inner Eden into the morass of left-brained didactics, analysis, over-mentalization, and stress. Now, I'm being given permission to move within, to my own sacred self. Peace, purity, love, contentment, and gentleness ease their way into my being.

We thirty-five students are divided up into small groups with one lead teacher in each. Our afternoons are spent in these clutches, processing the exercises and teachings of the day. We quickly and deeply bond in our empathy for one another and in wonderment for the new mind-body dimension we're entering. Basically, I spend this first intensive session purging my soul. There are dozens of times during exercises, when sharing with others, or in my room at bedtime, when the tears pour down my face as I let go of chunks of the heartbreak I've been carrying.

I mention to Kit that I feel self-conscious at times that I'm the only blubbering person here pouring out my heart.

"No, no, no, dear heart," she says. "All of us have pain and sadness to shed. You're in exactly the right place, doing exactly the right thing. You're healing and changing your realtionship between your emotions and your well-being."

"This feels like an ICU for emotional trauma," I whimper.

She smiles in compassionate understanding. "In some ways you could say so," Kit says, giving me a warm hug.

Over the next four days I learn that I'm so physically wrecked because of all that I've been carrying for years now. Negative self-beliefs, trauma, bottled-up anger, grief—it's all been too heavy to bear, so my body buckled to the Lyme disease. In turn, the crippling physical and emotional effect of Lyme itself has devastated my powers of hope and joy. Of course I'm exhausted and can't go on. And it's as plain as day to me now that I must learn a new way of being and relating in life, or I will never fully recover. I need to break out of the gridlock pattern of over-responsibility, worry, and the sublimation of my own needs. It strikes me as a new feeling that I actually want to care for myself.

By the end of this residential intensive I'm awash in emotion, shifts in energy awareness, and new ideas. A speck of peace has entered my solar plexus. The immediate nurturance I feel for this delicate seedling of new growth in me is like the love a mother feels for her brand-new baby. I protect it fiercely. I now understand healing in the context of a completely new paradigm.

It's a rather surreal moment when one of my new friends drops me off at my doorstep and I once again enter my small Victorian home. Somehow everything here looks just the same, but it all feels a tad different. It's not a bad thing, just an acute awareness. The ceiling is higher, the colors more vibrant. The sound of my voice seems to reverberate differently off the walls and sunlight falls on the crystal candlesticks with greater brilliance. Even Lucky's fur feels softer than ever.

"Hunter, do I look different to you?" I ask, as he cradles me in a big welcome-home hug.

"Let me see," he says, holding me back from him at arm's length, his hands bracing the sides of my shoulders.

"Well, your eyes look softer, and your face more relaxed. Something seems a bit brighter in you. But, honey, you still look just like you. Why?"

I want to tell him everything, but I am exhausted now and know that there will be plenty of time to share it all later.

"I feel different," I tell him, "better...in so many ways. But right now I just want to settle down, feel you and the house. Eli will be home shortly. Will you hold me?"

"Gladly," he says.

We nestle into the sofa together, my head resting on his sturdy chest, his arms wrapping me in an embrace of secure love. A tremor of energetic shiftings tingles through my nervous system. It is possible for me to heal—on so many levels. What an astonishing opportunity I am living!

Winter's Cloak

The arctic bite of December stings my bare hands as I wrap the carved front-porch pillars in spiraling strands of twinkle lights. Another Christmas descends on us, in our tiny home. I'm living small and simply, parceling out money from my dwindling savings to pay for rent and my mounting health-care bills. Eli's list to Santa Claus, tucked in to our mailbox, is long and diverse. iPod nano, nerf tag, and sculpting clay are just the tip of his wishes. How can I make his Christmas dreams come true with nothing much to shop with? The reality of my financial hardship is hitting me square between the eyes now, as I scrimp to manage presents under the tree.

I maneuver all my shopping online, as going to a store or a frantic mall is unthinkable with my still compromised energy. In fact, I barely ever drive my aged car at all. Every few weeks I ask Hunter to take it to his office, to give the engine a run. Otherwise my basic movement involves a walk to the video store or post office with Lucky. Others still do grocery shopping for me. "Day by day" is my present mantra, my lifeline to the Rife machine still humming.

Up goes another wee-sized Christmas tree, atop the coffee table. A PTO fir wreath adorns our front door. I play Nat King Cole carols ad infinitum, stirring our spirits upward. And, blessedly, Santa does arrive this year, bringing joy and a huge smile to Eli's face with a dozen boxes under the tree. Lucky even receives an enormous mesh stocking, chock-full of biscuits and rubber balls. Tenderly, I hug Eli good night as he heads to his father's home after our holiday dinner. My heart beats strong and sure within my chest, recanting to myself the many miracles of this past year. Energetically, I've made a huge deposit into my spiritual and emotional bank accounts with the momentous healing work I've undertaken at Stillpoint, and I just know the Rife technology is killing off the Lyme bacteria.

Another trip around the sun, I muse. *This year I'm happier and more whole. I'm not the person I used to be, but at least I feel some forward momentum.*

Just as my own three "wise ones"—Dr. Worthington, Dr. Pennell, Dr. Wu—have predicted, one year into treatment I can see and feel my progress. Still, I'm leery of the still likely presence of the Lyme cysto-spheres. Vowing to beat this disease, I hold fast and faithfully to all my treatment protocols: herbs, vitamins, homeopathy, Rife, acupuncture, walks, rest, and now my Stillpoint work. *I guess I'm discovering just how tenacious I can be.*

I finally get a follow-up MRI on the kidney. After a full day spent at Lahey Clinic under scrutiny by a renowned physician, I am given the freedom to not worry.

"This is likely nothing more than a blood-filled benign growth," I am told. "We'll rescan you yearly, but my belief is your kidney is fine."

This news is music to my ears at this point in my journey.

Since I left the Stillpoint intensive in early November, we've continued our schooling via weekly group telephone classes and at-home work sheets and exercises. My skills are rapidly developing. The partners in my small group circle are exceptional. We email one another regularly with supportive comments, questions, and dialogue. It feels like a true blessing to me. Just as the holidays of many spiritual traditions symbolize hope and healing at this time of the year, my own rebirth at Stillpoint is a tremendous and meaningful milestone. Along with all the bow-strewn boxes under our Christmas tree, I should've placed a drawing of my own heart, as I can feel it coming back to life.

Merry Christmas, Kim, I think.

The year 2007 enters in typical New Hampshire fashion with low-slung gray skies taped together by shallow light and icy temperatures. With the holiday spirit waning, January lumbers along in the single digits. Sometimes I walk out back after dinner and stare at the heavens above, stars strewn across the black canvas overhead in their lunatic array. An enormous, cone-shaped spruce tree looms beyond the barn roof, silhouetted by the floodlight from the realty office next door. I stand in the diluted light, gazing upon the reach of the tree's always still branches. This elder of my neighborhood trees somehow makes me feel peaceful and secure. I nod to it in honor.

I do miss my woodland home tucked in where thousands of kingly trees surrounded me with a sense of nurturance and magic. Yet life in town is not that bad. In fact, I mostly like it, in spite of the screeching brakes and siren wails. But on crystal-still nights like this, the snow squeaking under my footsteps in the dry air, I'm homesick for the majesty of the woods.

Drawing the muffler across my chin on this frozen winter's night, I feel a bit dejected in spite of the great gifts of 2006. I'm most definitely less ill than I was before. The fog in my head is receding and my energy has gained some, but I still have poor stamina and the aches and pains weigh me down. Plus, there are erratic migraines and I fight to fend off a faint depression. With what I am learning at school, I feel the pulse of healing, yet I am aware even now of the inner critic who looks for fault instead of offering encouragement.

"You're never going to get completely well again, Kim," its voice murmurs. *"Your glory days are over. Let's face it. You're now fat, lazy, broke, and sick. You'll never get back on your feet again. Your looks have faded and who wants to hang around a sickly middle-aged woman?"* Of course my fears run wild and I imagine Hunter leaving me, Eli moving to his father's full-time, me jobless and homeless, alone with no love or companionship. Weak and sick, I'd have to return to my family in Florida as a destitute.

I hate this mind game I play. Why do I beat myself up so? Why can't I be proud of the strides I've made in these two years? Instead of complimenting my resourcefulness and tenacity, I berate myself for not being more, sooner.

"Patience!" I say out loud in the night air.

I try to remind myself of how gentle and understanding I would be with my clients in this situation. I would praise their devotion to their cure, complimenting them for sticking with the homeopathic remedies, the acupuncture, the herbs, the Rife, their walks, and meditations.

In fact, I believe I would marvel at a client who exhibited such steady belief and consistency in his or her healing modalities. Instead I'm not nice to me. This is a bad tape I'm running in my head and all too often.

I return to the glow and warmth of my dwelling. Eli's TV shows chatter voices across the room. It's easy to feel the comfort I've created here. We live simply now, but all is well within. I remind myself of this. Lucky snuggles into his bed, next to the teeming warmth of the radiator. I draw the window shades and swallow my bedtime medicinals.

"Time for bed, Eli," I call out and we ascend the exceptionally steep stairs.

"Good night, Mommy," Eli's small voice calls to me from the next room.

"Good night," I say, "I love you, sweetheart."

As the cars shudder by in the snow-quilted street outside our home, I feel the peace of sleep wrapping me in arms of etheric diffusion.

Step-by-step, I remind myself softheartedly.

A Glimpse

Meredith holds Stillpoint's winter training on the balmy west coast of Florida. While I'm grateful for the opportunity to escape New Hampshire at this time of year, I'm actually frightened about making the long journey on my own. I still have trouble making it through the day without a nap, and my mental focus is sketchy. It feels impossible to me that I will physically hold up to both the travel and classwork. But I love what I'm learning so much that I'm crestfallen at the notion of not attending.

"Why don't I fly down with you, Kim?" Hunter offers. "That way I can handle the bags, the check-in, and getting you to the facility, and I can make sure everything there is comfortable for you."

"Really? You'd do that for me?" I ask, stunned awareness coloring my voice.

"You know I'd do anything for you, Kim," he says, smiling.

Soon enough, Hunter patiently guides me through the airport in a borrowed wheelchair. The trip is arduous, but nine hours later we make it to the hotel intact. I collapse on the polyester bedspread, wheezing myself to sleep in exhaustion and relief.

Classes begin the next day, and Hunter bids me a worried adieu. "Take your vitamins and herbs faithfully, Kim," he reminds me. "And make sure to get your sleep."

Just then my roommate happens to arrive, her laughter and energy filling the room in seconds. I can tell that Hunter senses Bette and I might well stay up yakking our way through the night.

"I promise to stay low-key, honey. Really," I reassure Hunter. "Bette's a nurse. She'll keep a good eye on me."

"Don't worry about her at all, Hunter," Bette says, her brown eyes sparkling with her mischief.

This doesn't reassure him at all, I'm sure.

"We'll do homework and be asleep by ten each night. No partying with the baseball players downstairs at all," she says, winking at me.

It just so happens our hotel is home to a major league Fantasy Week baseball camp while we are in residence. The place is crawling with middle-aged men and retired baseball players, here to play ball all week, while we sensitives are here to hone our intuition. It's quite a dichotomy of yin and yang.

"We'll be fine, Hunter. Don't worry. We'll avoid the testosteronis, really. We don't have time for anything other than class, meals, and homework anyway. I barely have time for my yoga."

"I know," he says. "Call me each night and let me know how you're doing. I'm going to worry about you, Kim." He hugs me close in goodbye at the elevator. "I'm not used to being so far away from you for so long. I've watched over your well-being for two years."

"I promise to keep to my routines and not overdo it," I say with a smile. "Don't worry, Papa Bear, I'm surrounded by so many healers, I'll have help if I need it. Plus I called on my eagle guide before we left New Hampshire."

He gives me one last hug, then slips onto the elevator, flashing me his "aw shucks" grin as the doors slide shut. Quickly, I return to my room, grab my books, papers, and air pad, and head off to class.

The days unfold with exhilarating purpose. Again, the healing exercises are profound. We're into the core of the metaphysical material now. Meredith instructs us how to garner salient intuitive insights about the collection of energy patterns and symptom states manifested within the body. I marvel at her understandings of the interconnectedness of thoughts or emotions and their physical consequences. It's exquisitely accurate information she conveys. Deciphering the language of intuitive pictures and impressions we receive about our own organs and glands during our practice exercises is fascinating to me.

"All right," says Meredith. "We're going to spend some time in our second chakra today and sense the patterns and messages there that pertain to the reproductive and urinary systems. Both are housed in the abdomen, which pinpoints the second chakra, a truly vital storehouse of energy. We rely on our urinary system to physically remove fluids and wastes from our body, as well as to energetically cleanse toxic emotions we've experienced, both personally and in relationship." She scans the room, sensing, before moving on, whether we're adequately absorbing this information.

"The reproductive system is one of cycles and balance. It represents renewal. We find a delicate balancing act between the past and the future, shedding energetic tethers from before and offering fertile ground to nurture our dreams. What we're working with here is an energetic message of conceiving our dreams and delivering them to fruition. Do we have any questions about this?"

A few hands go up and some discussion flows. We then delve into a practical exercise that helps us glean a more personal understanding about this chakra site of intimacy and connection, both in respect to our individual selves and to those we choose to share and co-create with. Out come the colored pencils and paper as Meredith has us enter a meditative practice.

While scanning my second chakra, I see a vivid picture in my mind's eye. It's of a twisted, tight knot on the right side, surrounded in a fiery red ball. It looks like it hurts. On the left portion of the scene, I find a soft, yellow, dawning light bathing a serene woman, who is standing next to a fawn. The feeling is of dreamy softness and peace. As we've learned in our classwork, the right represents the past, the left our future. I like where I'm going. I see alone time, reflection, a tender companion, less drama, and more creativity replacing the knotted, entwined, passionate fury of my past. I trust the images and the sense I have about them now, having spent months engrossed in interpretations of intuitive energy.

Having suffered through painful episodes of large ovarian cysts, it's stunning to learn the correlation between them and my unfulfilled life's dreams, entangled energetically in the knotty red ball. My disappointment over my failed marriages and the dashed dreams of having a large, laughter-filled family are lodged within my reproductive system, along with the residue of the torrid love affairs I crescendoed through. Of course these strong negative emotions could create some sorts of effects within me. The ovarian cysts and the knotty pains accompanying them are the energy I'm holding about my failed hopes and disillusionments. Our emotions and body are not disconnected.

The picture tells my story, I think to myself. That fiery red knot on the right is the lack of resolution from my past. To the left, I follow the gentle fawn into a soft morning light. I like the lovely woman standing there, at peace and in beauty. Realizing that this shows me my future, I actually feel my shoulders dropping down a few inches, my breathing relaxing, and my inner trust growing, realizing the worst is over and that a time of sanctuary awaits me. Knowing that I'm currently on the threshold of menopause, I sense that the fawn and contemplative woman I see represent the wiser, more tempered woman I'm emotionally growing into. In many ways it feels like a relief to me. The energy of tempestuous passion has been a lot to carry.

I open my eyes and scribble a sketch quickly, attempting to capture the essence of what I just saw and felt within. Meredith divides us up into groups of four, and we share our discoveries and questions, helping one another connect the dots. Some of our images are murky or confusing. It's helpful to share the images and feelings with others, learning how to decipher their meaning. In this intensive we've become familiar with a language that communicates the energetic patterns and messages of the chakras and what an organ is holding via the pictures that manifest.

"I've had eczema since I was kid," Lorraine conveys. "It's on the back of my scalp and ears. Who would've ever realized it all relates to the absolutely toxic emotional abuse I was subjected to growing up with my mean-tongued alcoholic father? I recall being terrified of him, the venom of my suppressed anger actually burning my scalp and ears. This eczema is the scalding energy I am still holding on to. I couldn't comprehend it all back then, but I see it clear as day now."

Similar scenarios unfold among my classmates as we unearth such pieces of self-discovery.

As predicted, Bette and I are up till all hours of the night, talking ourselves silly and laughing like high school kids. At one point I find myself hanging upside down off my bed, writhing in a gale of laughter over one of Bette's stories. The Fantasy Week ballplayers are essentially nonentities to us as none of us take to hanging out in the bar the way they do. One evening, though, when a few of us women do pop in for a glass of wine, the men are at the table like vultures, trying to ply us with drinks. It's amazing how strong our protective auric shields have become. The men veer away without incident.

A week later, I've shed a few light-years of karmic history and gained a much broader sense of my future. I feel lighter and brighter, less burdened, and much healthier. Most specifically, during this training module Meredith has helped each of us to hone in on our unique life's purpose. Instead of feeling conflicted and confused about my hopscotch life route, I am now excited to know that my most instrumental work is yet to come.

One morning, I see it all laid out before me. We are focusing on our third chakra, the energy site that covers the stomach area and the major linkage of organs there: the liver, stomach, gallbladder, pancreas, spleen, and intestines. Being what many sources refer to as the solar plexus, a place of gut reactions and our core of personal power and strength, this important chakra site is associated with our creative juices and resultant work in the world. In other words, the intention of our life's purpose and what we manifest is spawned from energetic alignment there.

Soon, I unearth a startling discovery that my treasured work as a homeopath is not the end-all-be-all of my life's work! The tears I shed over losing my career, back in the months of depressing illness at home on the sofa, need not sink me. During a powerful meditation and visualization exercise, I see myself happily at work in a pleasant space with a mountain view presiding in the west. There I sit, writing diligently in front of a large, sun-filled window, leafy green plants and warming colors nearby. I don't know exactly what it is I'm communicating, but it seems to be my way. I am reaching out and touching others. I like the looks of my future. I sense that it will be sunny and rewarding.

I hold on to this vision as I slip into the backseat of the taxicab, heading back to the icy cold of New England. I've learned so much, and we still have more training ahead of us.

Solo Journey

$\mathbf{B}$lue's brain cancer is advancing significantly and Hunter is deeply entrenched in the painful process of caring for her. The first rounds of experimental angiogenesis drugs last fall kept the now large brain tumor from growing any bigger, but the side effects are becoming too dangerous for Blue. Against Hunter's instincts and wishes, a more conventional and disfiguring chemo route is undertaken. The picture is not pretty, and brave Blue soldiers on with the most awe-inspiring patience and poise. She's the epitome of Zen mastery: be here, be now.

So many of us look on this fifteen-year-old girl with universal respect and great sympathy. It's obvious that she's physically uncomfortable, but she doesn't cry or whine, or even get angry. Blue's emotional temperance is enviable. We could all learn a great deal from this child.

Still, I've taken to shielding Eli from her disease. He knows that Blue is ill and getting special medicine, but it has rattled him deeply to see Blue's body becoming bloated and her hair falling out. Therefore, sadly, we no longer do things together. Lucky, though, goes for sleepovers at Hunter's apartment, bringing her comfort with snuggles and his ever-joyful energy. Nonetheless, Blue's health is seriously crumbling. Despair bores an ugly crevice into Hunter's soul. A haunted look invades his once-clear eyes and he sleeps fitfully, tangled in worries and consternations.

Nature's reassuring rhythms faithfully revolve, however, and wafts of spring showers scrub the air clean, leaving a sparkling bluish mist in their wake. Sprays of vivid jonquils bloom and the robin's cheerful song rekindles my hope. We celebrate both Eli's and Blue's birthdays in April, ages ten and fifteen respectively, and this school year I make it to poetry readings, open houses, and, surprisingly, even a class trip to a hilly sheep farm and a historical woolen mill. Though I take great care to maintain a steady routine, including my daily afternoon nap, my vigor has significantly improved from a year ago. The aging Jeep is even back on the roads more frequently. Dr. Pennell gives me the green light to resume swimming laps, as the Lyme and Epstein-Barr titres are improved. I'm elated.

It feels daunting, though, to drive twenty minutes up and back to the Olympic-sized pool at the rehab center where my fellow water rats churn through the lanes at blizzard rates. I elect to join the Wellness Center at our local hospital and attempt to swim against the current in the jet pool, knowing that it's barely frequented. Finding myself alone in this small turquoise square of water, I grapple with the roiling jet current, but eventually condition my body and mind, finding backstroke is the easiest solution. At first, five minutes is all I can handle. But, within a month's time, I work myself up to twenty minutes of rather vigorous swimming, my heartbeat thready and erratic at first but, ultimately, finding a more steady rhythm.

Dr. Wu assesses my pulses as much better. "Liver less tight, kidney chi stronger now, spleen still damp, but blood cracked no more," she reports at my monthly visit.

"Do you mean I'm getting better?" I ask.

"Yes, body much more balanced and strong. Emotions calmer, too. Still must not eat sugar or milk. Bad for spleen."

"I never eat dairy, but Hunter's a bad influence with the sugar," I tell her. "He loves dessert."

Dr. Wu smiles.

"Have fruit instead," she encourages me.

"Do you think the Lyme disease is better?"

"Yes, but you must still take herbs. Will take more time." With that she arranges a spiderweb of acupuncture needles across my body, leaving me dozing in the dimmed light for forty-five minutes of restoration.

I wander off on a windward journey amongst towering thunderheads and biblical rays of streaming golden light into a dreamscape of illusive dimension. It's funny how easy it is to slip into a trancelike sleep on her acupuncture table, my mind vacillating back and forth between asleep and awake. A hallway door creaks open. Voices from the waiting room trickle through the bruise-colored thunderheads. I let go of reality. Soon enough, I'm soaring high and wide above the Indian Ocean and off toward the South Sea Islands. Something tells me to come down to land. I try to but can't touch the earth. The outback of Australia looks torched and sizzling. I don't like its crusty face, though the beaches of the Great Barrier Reef seduce my playful, water-loving spirit. I realize I want to tell Hunter and Eli I'm going to New Zealand, but they're nowhere in sight. It's then that I realize I'm explicitly alone. This is my solo journey.

A strange feeling overtakes me. I'm untethered, afloat in the mighty altitudes like a big, beautiful hot air balloon, coasting serenely on transoceanic thermals. I want to land but feel too high actually to do it. Instead I keep drifting, languidly, loosely, dreamily, on a ribbon of wonder.

Where am I going? comes my thought.

No answer shows itself as I glimpse the coastline of Peru and the jutting mountaintops of the treacherous Andes. Skimming over the pointed peaks, my hand reaches out to touch the terrain, wanting to pat the fluffy body of a cocoa-brown llama or ground myself in one of the beckoning valleys. But on this hypnotic flight path I can't stop myself.

Soaring eastward and then north, I stare at the carpet of the thick Amazon jungle below. Howls and yaps, foreign tongues, and drumbeats float upward. As the Caribbean Sea comes into view, I can taste the coconuts and feel the tropical sun on my browning skin. The world begins to seem uncannily small and enormous all at once. The magnificence floods me.

Am I circumnavigating the globe? I wonder. *But why?*

I head off toward Europe. The Atlantic Ocean is wave tossed, the blue-gray seas cackling with the powerful wind. I had hoped to sail across the Atlantic one day in a sailboat. It was a life goal of mine years ago. Somewhere, on the verge of the Canary Islands, I snap awake on the acupuncture table. The dream blows off into the ethers, just as a haunted refrain slithers in on its tail.

"Perspective changes everything in life, dear." I remember the parting words of the mountain gnome years ago and let them seep into my fog-filled, sleepy mind. Both that mountain gnome and the eagle guide remind me to fly high above it all. *Why am I being reminded again to maintain an elevation? And isn't it interesting that I am alone on a mighty journey?* Mysterious and nonsensical both, these fleeting feelings and dreamy images converge somehow within me, registering as important in an intangible way.

How can I try to tell someone else that a dream or an unknown mountain trekker have influenced my reality? They'll think I'm too far out, that the Lyme disease has affected my brain function. It's hard to convince others of the validity of intuitions or images when we've all been conditioned to accept only the black-and-white literal data of science. But with all that I'm learning at Stillpoint, I'm coming to understand how direct and accurate intuitions and conscious visualizations typically are.

Dr. Wu returns, removing the delicate needles, retaking my pulses, and sending me on my way. I can't shake a nagging sense of unsettledness that has crept in, however.

I'm evolving, higher and more broad in my view, I think. *Something important is surfacing.*

Another Avian Teacher

After a particularly heavy outpouring of maple sap this season, the sugaring shacks finally squelch their billowing trails of smoke. The days are lengthening once again. Stronger now than a year ago, my stamina obviously enhanced, I get myself outdoors, with my easel and paints, tapping into my creative energy. This time the outing feels more feasible and real. I actually manage to mix my palette with swift ease. I am fortunate to live in a location with such lavish scenery and endless painting opportunities. They urge me onward to capture the beauty.

Today, while painting en plein air on a backwoods New Hampshire roadside, I watch a great blue heron stepping with measured patience along the pond's perimeter. On tall, twiggy legs she moves through the water like a high-stepping majorette in freeze-frame motion, keen eyes alert for fish, neck feathers afloat in a nimbus shawl. I remain motion-less, afraid to move a muscle and perhaps frighten her away.

Suddenly, the bird plunges her long beak into the glassine water and, after a quick flip of her head, a wriggling fish slips down her throat. She remains stock-still. Silently, on shallow breath, I marvel at this masterful fisher's confident skill and quiet grace. Her exquisite mark-ings and noble beauty are readily camouflaged amidst the needle-fine marsh reeds.

Across the pond, in a flat-bottom skiff, a red-shirted fisherman casts his line. Crisp, starched clouds drift across the lazy blue sky. I take in the scene, absorbing every detail. An unexpected dog's bark breaks the moment of suspended serenity and the heron takes flight. I watch her ascend in a few strong wingbeats, over the pond, those crooked stalk legs now trailing in a more refined posture. She rounds the point of this marshy cove and is out of sight.

I realize in these pensive moments that the heron, too, can teach me some lessons. I admire her patience, her ability to move so slowly, with great care and intention, and think about all my grumbling and complaining over these years of stillness and solitude. I've longed to be out in the world doing so many things instead of being quiet and contemplative at home. But looking at the heron, I reflect. *She's the embodiment of stillness, presence, and grace. I marvel at her ability to live her life in such a way. Why can't I think of myself as living like a heron?*

I take stock: I can move, though slowly. I can curl and twist, bend and roll. I walk my dog up and down hills. I swim in the ocean and lakes. I'm not in a wheelchair, as some people are. I must be grateful for what I have.

I know that I'm not the only one who struggles with feelings of self-pity. How many thousands of others are sidelined by the debilitating effects of Lyme disease? Multitudes hover on sofas and beds like me, too drained to do anything more than just the bare necessities of daily functioning. In fact, some can't even do that. Anyone living with chronic illness that imposes severe limitations must experience similar feelings of disappointment, frustration, fear, sadness, and envy. I am not alone.

Yet it is a challenge to live solely in the state of being; being still, being with one's feelings, being with just one's inner self. We crave life's distractions. Ours is a society addicted to constant motion and stimulation: jobs, households, kids' schedules, and electronics all running in a synchronized manner. Do we have a place or time to cultivate stillness and self-reflection anymore? Is it illness that has taught me to turn within?

It's okay that I got sick, I suddenly realize. If the Lyme hadn't taken me down so radically, I wouldn't have learned about stillness. I would not have discovered my enormous capacity to endure. I would not have embraced this deeply contemplative place within my own being. I might never have made it to the Stillpoint School. And, most important, I might never have made the changes needed to follow my own life's purpose and discover the true energy of healing. Instead, I would've kept running furiously ahead, doing what I was trained to do: achieve more than the generation before me.

I'm breaking the pattern. Of course I feel inept and inadequate. No wonder it has scoured me so to lose the emblems of American ideals: career success, marriage, home, health, and savings. Remarkably, it has taken me all this time to discover that I don't have to do it that way. I can still be a wonderful person with an entirely different set of valued assets. Fortitude, creativity, loving compassion, and wisdom are just as meaningful as a steady income, a cohesive marriage, and a well-funded IRA, if not more so.

These years in my hermitage have not been wasted. I see now how much I've grown. In an unexpected way, this passage has given me the experience of retreat. The hours spent in meditation, prayer, contemplation, and stillness have brought me into the deepest chambers of myself. I've intimately tasted the good and the bad within. It has been fantastically difficult at times, wrenching even. The lovely heron reminds me, though, that grace and beauty reside within me, too. The inner peace I've discovered can never be underestimated. I've gained immensely in depth, breadth, and—like the mountain gnome told me—perspective.

Suddenly I feel very dizzy. The treetops begin to look a bit wobbly to me. I lie down on the ground, fatigue descending. It feels different from being plainly tired. Something visceral inside me is radically shifting. An entirely new paradigm is emerging within me. My orientation to living, achieving, and believing is being altered by my own personal earthquake.

Life has asked me to change. How fiercely I've been resisting this. No more mastering mountains or thundering through divorce proceedings. Instead the poetic great blue heron will inspire me. I've become steady and still. Watchfulness and wisdom are taking root within me. I'm moving forward, like her, with purpose, awakening.

Heartsong

Summer often arrives in a cavalcade of steamy surprise in New Hampshire. I miss Long Island's extended unveiling of the blossoming dogwoods and apples, azaleas and tulip trees. In these parts, we're dipped in hideous swarms of blackflies, pelted with deluges of rain, and, in the flip of a coin, jolted into ninety-degree scorches. This year is no different. I pack for my final week of training, putting tank tops and sundresses into my suitcase. Of course the Rife is in tow, but I don't include the air pad for rest time, assuming I'll hold up all day now on my own.

Arriving at Stillpoint we're all abuzz in camaraderie and chatter. The friendships I have knitted here are rich and treasured, my bond to each classmate unique. It feels wonderful to be back with my new family of friends. Nine months into our training now, we've each spent an enormous amount of time steeped in daily meditations and healing prayers. The homework assignments and phone classes have bridged the gaps in terms of keeping our intuitive skills honed and giving us a clear grasp of the metaphysical dynamics between our bodies and minds. But nothing can replace the experience of gathering together here in residence.

I open my eyes after an hour-long meditation and sermon, gazing on a roomful of prayer shawls hugging shoulders in casual comfort. Our quiet journey toward the soul's center casts a certain glow of palpable reverence. The feeling is one of acceptance and trust. "Steady, steady, steady" is a favorite mantra of Meredith's. Over and over she reminds us in her teachings, her writings, and in private counsel to steady our runaway emotions. Here we all sit in unison, hands placed over our hearts, breathing in and out in a conscious and steady rhythm. I feel the sure tempo of my heartbeat. The wooden floor is solid beneath my feet. Rain taps on the roof. Within this room I sense a certain peace, a quiet grace, and a profound degree of respect amongst us all. Deeply centered, steady within my core and calm inside my heart, I'm open and eager for the massive volume of information Meredith will surely download on us today.

A tone of melancholy pervades this final week, though, as we know that many of us will not cross paths again physically for a long time. Still, those of us wishing to pursue certification as intuitive healers will continue another two months afterward as interns, honing our skill sets and techniques. Being fully vested in the palpable mechanics of this fascinating work, I, of course, elect to further my studies. I'm saying good-bye to this glorious group of wise and gifted individuals, though a smattering of us will remain in contact throughout the summer. This feels right to me.

Stillpoint tradition includes a graduation ceremony. We learn via our small-group teachers that the class selects a thank-you gift for Meredith in recognition of all that she so generously gives to us. One evening we converge in two classmates' room to select our communal gift. Our brains reel and turn, conjuring up the most meaningful choice.

After much deliberation, a single yet perfect notion is agreed on. We'll put together a booklet of our individual heartsongs, which Meredith helped us create a few months prior. Creative and personal, they're filled with the beauty of self-knowing. The icing on the cake is that we will include an individual photo of each graduate next to his or her heartsong.

Just before we leave the meeting a suggestion surfaces that we need to select a person to make the presentation and speech at graduation. But how do we elect just one from all of us? Scanning the broad array of faces and talents surrounding me, I am surprised to hear three or four voices in agreement.

"Kim, Kim. The person who should make the presentation is Kim." All eyes are looking at me.

"What, me?" I say in disbelief. "No, Terri is doing all the computer work on this project; it should be her."

"No, I'm not a good speaker. I don't like standing up in front of a crowd. All this year it has been you, Kim, who has repeatedly shared perceptive words and insights. You understand this work so well. You communicate so clearly in a way that is so inclusive and kind."

"Most important, you healed the most dramatically amongst us all," Laura says.

Many heads nod yes and voices confirm her opinion.

I am both shocked and honored. "Really?" I ask. "I thought I always sounded so harebrained and sketchy, so emotional."

"Not ever," Terri says. "You're astute and thoughtful, and so poised."

"Wow. I guess I never saw myself that way, with all the drama and crying I've been dealing with."

"Precisely. It's your honesty and bravery that has inspired so many of us," Jonathan says. "And look at you now, upright and strong, healthy and vibrant. A year ago you had to lie down most of the class. Now you walk the trails up and down the mountainside. Your healing has been dramatic."

I catch my breath and swallow hard. Could my friends really be right? I guess I have made huge progress. It still stuns me. Thinking for a few moments, I recognize the outpouring of support these dear people are showing me. Their love and respect touches me.

"Please, Kim," Jonathan says again. "You're the best one to do this for us. We know you'll find the perfect words of thanks for Meredith."

I feel a bit scared but also proud. Of course I want to help everyone to do a good job.

"Okay," I agree. "But I need to practice my speech with one of you."

"No problem," says Bette.

We scurry to our rooms to type, draw, shoot photos, and print. I copy over my heartsong, using my best penmanship to ready it for Terri:

. . . Waves wash me,
Sun restores me,

Surfsong fills me.
Tenderly, my rhythms weave together.
Restored and cleansed,
I bring my Self to wholeness.

The last night here at Stillpoint, Hunter comes to join me. We decide to take a soak in the palatial, twenty-foot hot tub, bubbling in froth and sprinkled by a waterfall. I float on my back, gazing up into the mirrored ceiling of the geodesic dome. I see myself, arms and legs extended in starfish fashion, the heat and water enveloping me in a womb of safety. Hunter twirls me very slowly in the water, cradling my head in one hand. A feeling of bliss wraps its tender arms around me. All the difficult emotions and physical pains that have surfaced in this year of intense spiritual discovery evaporate into the soothing water. It is like a baptism. I feel the trickle of salty tears as I let go of my past and the wayward patterns. Gazing up into the dome above, I search into the skeleton of the heavens for guidance along my life's course. All I see are the rippling pale-blue water, my body's starfish formation, and Hunter's steady presence.

There are no answers given. I hear the words inside myself. As much as I want someone or something to tell me how to proceed with my life, to tell me if I'll ever really be healthy again, I realize that I must find my own way and honor my intuition.

Commencement

The next morning a gossamer breeze skims over my bare shoulders as I walk amid the shady pines, their soft, fallen needles padding my footfall. I've become attached to this early morning stroll down the wooded mountainside trail, past the joe-pye weed and Queen Anne's lace, en route to the carriage house classroom. As the seasons have evolved, so have I.

With each breath I take, I know deep within myself that my efforts here at the Stillpoint School have changed my life forever. My classmates are correct: my spirit has been mended in a very deep way. An entirely new consciousness and language have opened up to me now that I understand the intimate metaphysical relationship between emotions and illness. Intentionally incorporating a union between intuitive knowing and the practicalities of Western science–based medicine, Meredith has taught us that two hands working together are more capable than just one. By changing my conscious thoughts, I have changed my own body's neurochemical reactions and consequent well-being. My hope is that I can share these newfound tools with others in need.

Stepping inside the chambers, roses and candles meet my eyes, and glorious music fills the air. A small gallery of friends and family has come for our graduation ceremony. I see Hunter in the second row. My classmates and I gather together, smiles passing between us. This experience has made us warriors of the spirit. We believe in one another implicitly. I think to myself that this curriculum should be entitled "Inward Bound" for all the dare and trust, challenge and growth it calls forth.

The group stands in a large circle, Meredith at the top, backdropped by the enormous fieldstone fireplace. With butterflies batting about inside my stomach, I break from my position and go stand face-to-face with our teacher. It's time for me to offer our collective gratitude. Our gift is in my hands. Taking a huge gulp of air, I drop my anxious energy down into my belly and deliver the speech I have carefully prepared.

I speak of our wondrous year, the remembrance of this firelit chamber on initiation eve, and how I felt akin to Dorothy in *The Wizard of Oz*, far from home and seeking a direction. I acknowledge the deep journey we have all taken toward our heart's center and the tremendous value of this work and of our treasured teacher. Heartfelt and poignant, my words ring in the rafters, reflecting not only my own sentiments, but also those of all my classmates.

By the end of my address, tears loll on Meredith's eyelashes and mine. Small chokes of air heave from some classmates behind me. I hand our mentor her gift and then bow deeply in gratitude. Carefully, she unwraps the paper, finding first a scrumptious floral prayer shawl in rose-and-green symphony. She loves it. Then she has the book of heart-songs in her hand. We know from her deep, rich laugh and exclamations of delight that our choice is a great success. I peer over her shoulder, gazing on the unique writings and photos on each page, some with sketches and artifacts attached. It truly is a testimony to the magic of what Meredith has winnowed from all of us.

By the time we each receive our certificates and white silk Tibetan prayer shawls, a great golden hush bathes the room in a plentiful grace. I walk out into the boulevard of summer a completely different person than I was a year ago, eminently more happy and proud, and filled with the promise of new tomorrows.

Metamorphosis

I swim in the pond daily now. Slipping back and forth through the olive-green waters, I count out my makeshift laps along the buoyed rope line at the back of the designated children's swimming area. Powder-blue skies transmute to quilted gray clouds and return anew, freshly laundered and sparkling, one day to the next. Breathe and blow, breathe and blow, circling arms stretching up to the heavens and forging down into the hidden depths. The progression of my healing grows with each mile conquered as I swim away from the choking haze of illness and depression.

Canvases clutter our little cottage: farmyard vignettes, sun-soaked meadows, and auburn ridgelines dipped in purple sunsets, all tracing my days en plein air. How fantastic it feels to be back at the easel after three years of collapse. My goal is to have enough work ready to exhibit in the Art Colony Studio Tour in October.

I'm working hard now, physically by building up my stamina with exercise, emotionally by maintaining my spiritual meditative practice, and creatively by painting when I can. I don't dare let down any of the trusted health-care modalities. The blood tests show improvement. The Lyme is abating, although the Epstein-Barr virus will not recede, still active in my system. Homeopathic remedies are indispensable, easing me through a week of neck pains or a spell of the blues. Without question the Rife machine is my great hero. Four days per week I faithfully use it, code 26 humming in my palms, driving out lingering *Borrelia* bacteria and cystosphere hatch-outs. I have added Epstein-Barr frequencies to the repertoire now also.

In spite of all my efforts, I still have unwell spells. For no specific reason, a day dawns where I feel cloudy and weak, barely able to make it out the door.

Hunter encourages me to hold on. "It will pass," he promises. "In a couple of days you'll feel better. Just wait and rest. You'll see."

Sure enough, he's correct. A few extra doses of mitochondrial support or quercetin and I awaken to better mental clarity and less hollow breathing. The spell passes off like a summer shower traipsing across the hilltops.

I have many wondrous days out on the golf course this summer with Eli. With little to sink my teeth into in terms of my own worldly accomplishment, I'm finding a vicarious pleasure in helping Eli develop his skills. He is quite gifted at golf, actually, and it tickles me to no end when he stubbornly resists advice from anyone else, insisting, "Mommy is my coach."

Eli and I talk and laugh together in the cart, jostling over the bumpy paths.

"Head down, don't cock your wrist so much," I remind him. "Bring your hips through."

I watch with pride as he deftly chips a ball up onto a choice green or gracefully finesses a beautiful one-hundred-fifty-yard drive over a gully. We're two peas in a pod, reveling under the open skies. And, like my mountain ascent and painting pleasures, our golf outings inspire me toward a happier and healthier place.

Hiking has returned to my life, too, though I have yet to tackle a mountain peak. Our region boasts an endless bounty of beautiful trails around ponds and lakes, behind old, fallow farmsteads, and along relic logging roads. Once again, I find my way back into the woods, now merely as a visitor and well sprayed with insect repellent, but still in awe of its splendor. I inhale the soft aroma of the velvetine fern fronds as Lucky and I sit side by side on a moss-cushioned boulder, a stream running hastily along. My trips into the woods are cherished moments still, tuning my heartstrings into a balance not attainable at home or amid others. The solitude, textures, and elements have such a power over me. Humankind cannot induce the calmative effects nature does. Here, I'm reminded of New Hampshire's special gifts of wilderness retreat.

In spite of the loveliness I still find on these woodland trails, I now note a peculiar new awareness within me. It shocks me the first couple of times I sense this feeling, but many outings later it is still present. As odd as it may sound, I no longer feel at home in the woods. Something has radically shifted within me. Whether it's trauma from the horrific Lyme experience, association with my tumultuous married years there, or the real fact that I've moved on in some energetic way, the woods no longer wrap me in the same seductive arms of delight they once did. The years of horseback rides on shadowy paths, the childhood summers of backpacking, the mystical yearnings to surrender into the woods' rich, beckoning beauty all fall away from me like an orange rind from the fruit. Somehow, I don't need its endless secrets anymore now that I have come to explore the depths within.

I stand, peeled and denuded, comfortable in my own skin, freed from so much of my past, a new person. I've come to realize that healing is so much more than ministering to the physical body, its chemistry, hormones, and organ functions. As a human being and as a health-care practitioner, I have evolved profoundly. I have leaned that the heart and spirit require just as much attention and care as an open gash. An emergency can occur on any plane, yet both the body and soul are impressively resilient.

Powwow

There is one place, hidden deep in the woods, where I still love to go. Ducking under the draping hemlock veil, one steps onto a buttressed granite knoll, spattered with mossy pocks, overlooking pristine teal water. Although small in dimension, this pond is bountiful in beauty. I've showed it to less than a handful of special people in my life, as I dare not spread word of its existence and spoil its purity. To me it's a sacred space. This open altar commands a stunning view and an even more stunning sense of knowing peace. Here, I can sit for hours and contemplate life, the miracle of such beauty, or the changing wisps of vagrant cloud strands that flounce and stray overhead.

Now, on a perfect, late September morning, Hunter, Lucky, and I jostle the trusty Jeep over the unnamed dirt roads to the unmarked entry point into this hidden sanctuary. It's a place you come to by sight markings, not by GPS. After making the fourth turn down a series of rutted old back lanes, we park on the woods' edge next to a tractor-sized, lichen-encrusted boulder. The calls of songbirds ring in the air. Lucky is off in a flash on the scent of some woodland creature. Hunter and I grab water bottles and a satchel of fruit for our one-mile hike in.

Up a slight incline and past a crumpled stone wall, we proceed southwest, following the surprisingly wide pathway. It stretches a solid twenty feet across, an old road of some sort. Strong deciduous trees and younger saplings make up this forest, dotted with clusters of white pine and hemlock. This is not a particularly old forest. In fact, it's considered rather young, perhaps fifty to sixty years old at most. Occasionally, we spy a thick, twisted old wolf pine with its numerous upper trunks reaching for the sky.

Each time we walk this trail to the secret pond, we catch another glimpse of information, helping us dream our way into the pond's past. Our biggest curiosity always is the sharp-edged, flat-surfaced stone canal on the road's last downhill turn, at the pond's north perimeter. The water here is dark brown and stagnant, dotted with green clots of duckweed and floating sticks. Damselflies and broad-footed water bugs gather on the surface, dancing along in movement. Hunter and I have decided this now magical pond was once a rock quarry, accounting for its significant clarity and depth, considering its rather diminutive size. The canal was where the cut rock slabs were likely "floated" out on logs and loaded on ox-drawn carts, to be transported to the nearby train tracks, merely a couple of miles away and long gone, destroyed in the hurricane of '38. Now, the pond and its history lie placid and sleepy.

Far off to the south, trailing in on a warm breeze, I hear a festive tumble of sound, a timbre of pitch, drumlike and resonant. Between thumps, a kind of whooping catches my ear. Lucky stands alert, too, his large corgi ears pricked upright.

"Do you think someone's having a party?" I ask Hunter.

"Maybe so," he replies. His hearing is less acute than mine and he strains to catch the sounds.

I listen for a bit as we turn off from the open patch of grass at pond-side and head into the last stretch of deer path that will swing us along the granite stone ledges, up to the veil of hemlock and the stone hillock I love to sit on.

Just as I reenter the forest, a jolt blasts through my mind. "Hunter," I cry, "those are drums from the Native American powwow! I saw the signs in town yesterday. Let's go on the way home."

We spend an hour at the pond in a dreamy reverie. Hunter and I chat while relishing our snack, our bodies stretched out on the ancient granite. Lucky wades into the inviting water. I join him, socks and shoes shed. Knee-deep in the purifying beauty, I turn to see tears rolling down Hunter's cheeks. I feel the cloistering weight of his pain. Outwardly,

Hunter appears as implacable as these formidable rocks, yet I know that his heart has absolutely fractured as Blue has deteriorated in these past months. Returning to his side, I lay my cool hand on the back of his neck. His head slacks forward in fatigue. A terminally ill child is too tragic a burden for anyone to bear. In silence, breathing in unison, I sit beside Hunter, my right arm entwined with his, doing what we do best together: bearing witness to one another's life pain.

When the time feels right, we hike back to the Jeep and bump our way into the campground powwow site. The place is swarming with people, tents and teepees, booths, and food. Hunter and I wander amid the massive assortment of trinkets, feathered headdresses, painted leather pouches, carved fetishes, and pretty silver jewelry. Drums and flutes, chants and dances color the periphery. The festivities are under way in the large, roped-off central arena of an open meadow. Soon enough we make our way to the sidelines, securing a spot to watch and take in the ritual. My senses are filled with voices and languages I'm not familiar with, but the drums soothe me in a steady, primal way. I feel them in the core of my belly, filling me up and rounding out my heart. Unexpectedly, Hunter's cell phone goes off and he takes the call, a stern and gloomy expression dropping over his face.

"I have to leave right now," he says in a clipped tone. "Blue's being rushed to Boston by ambulance. Her breathing is failing. This could be bad, Kim. The last week has been hellish; her body can take only so much."

"I know, sweetheart, I know." I wrap him in a big hug, feeling his concern and fear. We turn from the crowd and race to the car.

"Eli is coming home in a few hours," Hunter says. "You stay with him and I will call you from Boston Children's when I know more."

"I'm here for you in all ways," I tell him, anxiety seeping into my chest.

Hunter drops me outside my little home and heads off into the maze of roads leading the eighty-five miles to Boston. I go inside and light a candle, placing it in front of Blue's sixth grade class photo, her big brown eyes looking out at me, calm and knowing. I now comprehend the vision that came to me that day on the acupuncture table. A high perspective is demanded of me now more than ever. I must maintain my eagle vision and inner truth. Life is both precarious and precious.

On day three of his bedside vigil in Boston, I beg Hunter to come home to New Hampshire for an overnight respite. "You need a good meal," I tell him. "Not to mention a bed to sleep in and a hot shower. Please drive up tonight."

"No, Kim," he says. "I don't care if I never eat or sleep. Blue is so critical. I must be with her."

I can feel his pain and commitment and I know that he needs to be cared for, too.

"Just twelve hours for recharge will help you through the days ahead," I reason. "I'm cooking pot roast for you right now. Please get in the car. I'll take care of you, honey."

There's silence on the phone line for a few moments. I feel him reeling in exhaustion.

Later, Hunter sleeps in my arms like a war-torn soldier, a dank fear radiating from him even in slumber.

Transitions

A few nights later, Hunter's friend ferries me down to the hospital. In Ron's sturdy green pickup, we descend from the New Hampshire foothills, weaving through the decrepit Massachusetts mill towns. I watch the laquered periwinkle sky mute to an onyx glow, my heartbeat quickened by tension. Ron and I emerge into the thick of Boston's traffic, the loopy network of streets causing us to miss the Boston Children's Hospital exit and end up going the wrong direction on a one-way street. Ron eventually skims his vehicle into the parking garage, the heavy-duty kayak roof racks missing the overhead girders by mere inches.

Hunter meets us in the hospital lobby. He looks like hell, sleepless smudges under his eyes, stubby beard growth, and an abyssmal sadness hooding him. I glide into his arms and his sobs seep into my collar. His perspiration reeks of ketones, with an overlay of that nauseating pharmaceutical hospital smell. My heart breaks for his pain.

A pall hangs over Blue's darkened room despite the bounty of flowers, cards, and cheerful photos. She is unconscious, her only movement a subtle flickering under her eyelids and a chesty breathing. Blue's loved ones surround her, wailing tears. I pull Hunter out into the hallway and ask him if I can do some energy work on her.

"I sense that her spirit is weighted down," I tell him. "She's struggling to ascend, but is worried about leaving you all. Can you reassure her that you're okay and let me open her chakras?"

In bleary sadness, Hunter nods and we reenter the room together. I say a prayer to Blue. Tenderly, I weave a web of sacred energy over her body, at her seven chakra sites, as I learned to do in my intuitive training. Just as I finish the release, Blue opens her eyes, gazes directly at me, and smiles. I give her my greetings and blessings. She smiles at her father and then slips back into the netherworlds. Our fated lifetime together has reached its end. I'm deeply touched that she chose to see me this one last time, hearts woven across the veil.

We lose gentle Blue in the dawning hours of September 30, 2007. Her fifteen-year battle with cancer is over. The final days and hours have broken down the heavily reinforced walls of Hunter's heart. He becomes completely unraveled, a broken man—and understandably so. Crying and aching in a drowning grief, he wanders aimlessly, ungrounded and unshaven, in crumpled clothes.

The pendulum swing of life is not random. Blessedly, at the time of Blue's passing my strength and well-being are at a recent peak. I'm able to be completely present and available for Hunter. As he so tenderly cared for me in the darkest hours of my Lyme disease ordeal, I in turn now minister to his overwhelming pain. I bathe him, feed him, and rock him in my arms in the depth of night. With family and friends in attendant support, we prepare for a memorial service for Blue. Time stands still in the slow-motion days of suspended disbelief following her passing. Hunter is dangerously bereft. I watch him with my eagle eye.

October 5 dawns with a ripe streaming glory of autumn sunshine. Hearts are heavy in our home, relatives gathering, friends attending, holding so much of Hunter's grief and the vacuum of Blue's disappearance from our world. For five days, Hunter's childhood friend Ben, his brother Clark, and I have held close to one another, never leaving Hunter alone for more than a few minutes. His wrenching heartache makes him fragile and raw, but the four of us weave together in a safety net of care and love.

As the frenetic whirl of preparations mounts, we each feel pressured and taut, yet filled with a reverence, too. The Indian summer day soars into the eighties. Shirts are being ironed, notes scribbled, phone calls returned. I decide to take one last swim at the pond before the service, a daring move in frigid October waters.

The water glistens in shimmering reflections of brilliant oranges and wine reds. Standing knee-deep, a tad shivery, I realize that this swim is for Blue, as she so joyfully adored the water. It will be my gesture of honoring her. Plunging in, heart lurching with the cold, I open my eyes to see the sandy floor, tawny and soft, a few minnows to my right, and the greening depths luring me farther in. I swim strong and fast, straight into the center of the pond. It's brisk, invigorating, and serenely elegant out here. Floating on my back, gazing into the azure above, I hold my mind steady with an image of Blue, her brown eyes and eternally childlike smile, looking straight back at me. I see us swimming together in the rushing waters of the Swift River, wriggling our way on tummies through the Lost River Caves, and advancing hand in hand into the frothing waters at Montauk Beach on a perfect August day a few summers ago. As these memories swell through me, I sense a peace, a knowing, a silent nod inside, that Blue is free and unchallenged now in the spirit plane. The words *resting now* float into my mind. It soothes me to feel this message about her. I swim slowly and intently back to shore.

Outside the classic, spired New England village church, arms enfold us again and again in the gilded light as we make our way up the stone steps, past the overflowing crowd, and into the front pew. Hunter's hand trembles in mine. The grief swarms in rivers around my head, tears flowing from everyone's eyes. We all miss Blue. Memories are shared of this special girl, her tremendously brave and accepting spirit, and the gifts of trust, mindfulness, and patience she so miraculously taught us all in her brief fifteen years. The music is especially perfect and Hunter's heartfelt a cappella rendition of "Amazing Grace" goes right to the marrow.

At the service's end, Hunter and I step out into the welcoming rays of autumn's splendor, riotous colors branching forth on the weathered maple trees. I'm reminded that life begins and ends over and over, season after season, life after life, time after time. As four-hundred-plus people emerge from the church, moving down to us on the front lawn, the love pours and bathes over us, with each handshake, hug, and moment shared. It's all so beautiful, so enriching, so poignant. We are touched deeply by all who have come to remember Blue and to support us and the rest of her family in this time of transformation.

In late October, holding Hunter's quavering hand, I walk him in the evening dusk to Meredith's side for a retreat program at Stillpoint. Slowly, the healing of his own splintered heart begins.

Winter Solstice

In December 2007 a significantly new chapter dawns. With help on a mortgage loan from my eternally loving, aging father, I buy a lovely home. My "Doris Day" ranch is situated in a pretty neighborhood on the lip of town. It's not in the woods but on a remarkable piece of land once called Highland Meadow. I immediately sense the solidity, comfort, and joy of this house, custom-built forty years ago for a family of four. It's sun-filled and centered on a broad open lawn, graced by beautiful maples and a stately giant Norwegian blue spruce standing sentinel. We even have a wintertime mountain view. The energy here is special.

We move in a few days before winter solstice, the snow swirling in a comforting downy peace, my heart pinwheeling with the humming knowledge that my true healing is here. I have come home, full circle, after a trying and often frightening journey, only to discover the richest strength lies within my very own self.

After many days of moving, over one hundred boxes lie stacked in the new house's basement and garage. Where to begin in the chore of unpacking? Blithely, I wander into the garage, stand amid the towering cardboard array, and randomly reach out, selecting a moderate-sized box to begin with. I carry it back into the lovely, sun-speckled living room, the light from the western picture window casting a warm glow on the broad brick fireplace and stark, empty mantel.

I don't recognize my numbering system or handwriting on the box top. Somehow, it's vaguely familiar to me, though. I slit open the packing tape binding with scissors. Sifting through the neutral white stuffing paper, my fingers feel a hard object. It's not too heavy. I pull it out. My breath catches as my eyes take in the exquisite blue-and-white porcelain China vase. It was my mother's. I haven't seen this item in many years. It was packed away in my basement, safe from toddler's reach, box top numbered in my sister's hand.

"Are you here?" I ask, all the while sensing that she is. "Do you like my new house?"

There is a perfect peace. I feel Patricia's magnificence, and a rush of warmth. Her dazzling smile flashes before my eyes. Alert, yet in a stunned silence, I sense the fresh palette of this completely empty house, no signs of life or the prior owner around me. The cupboards are bare, the walls unadorned, the air sweetly quiet, my furniture due in tomorrow. I am aware that this home is an utterly blank canvas.

I can create another future, I think to myself. *I'm starting over, once again.*

I walk back to the garage and randomly select a second box from a different section, another corner completely. I bring it in and open it. This time I pull out a stunning pair of marigold yellow and buttermilk blue French candlesticks, pieces my mother treasured and knew I, too, admired. At the bottom of the packing paper is her calico-covered box of handwritten recipes on lined, aging index cards. I see Mother's distinctive loopy Palmer penmanship:

> To my darling daughter and wonderful hostess, Kim. May these longtime favored recipes bring you many happy meals. I love you forever and ever, Mother.

I feel her love pouring into me. By now my cheeks are wet with tears as I gingerly place my mother's long-hidden belongings on my vacant mantel. The house is serenely still.

"Thank you, Mother," I whisper. "There's no place like home!"

With that, the door flies open, and Eli and Lucky come bouncing in, brimming with life, energy, and unfathomable joy. My heart swells to the very top, relishing my many blessings in this incredible journey toward healing. Undeterrable Hunter follows the two inside, carrying an armful of firewood and beaming a big smile.

"How do you like it here, honey?" he asks.

"It's perfect. Absolutely perfect!"

Life Circles

I am well now. My energy has returned. I swim a mile with ease and daily in the pond during the summer months. I dance and twirl just as Hunter told me I would, six horrific summers ago, wracked by the shrapnel of Lyme. But now the *Borrelia* are killed off, and the Epstein-Barr is held at bay. Dr. Pennell has run tests several times over the past two years, finding my Lyme values to be excellent on the CD 57 test, signifying that my body is not actively "fighting" the Lyme bacteria.

"Of the dozens of patients I have treated with chronic Lyme disease," Dr. Pennell says, "you're the only one, Kim, who has beaten it without using antibiotics. I had come to think it wasn't possible with the herbs."

"I believe that the Rife and homeopathy supports were the mainstay," I tell him. "I still keep on a weekly Rife-maintenance schedule, along with a lifetime low dose of cat's claw, too. I figure if in five years we still find me to be in the safe zone, then I'll drop the vigilance. I fought so hard to reclaim my life; I dare not let it slip away from me again."

"Your positive mind-set and self-belief surely helped, too."

My illness taught me many lessons. Moderation, balance, and time for solitude are still critically important, and my morning meditation, prayers, and journaling have become a permanent part of my repertoire. Some form of daily exercise is also a staple, whether it be swimming, walking, yoga, or dancing. I need to maintain social connections, too, being a consummate extrovert, or my spirits wilt. One of the most significant gifts born from this experience is the access I've gained to my creative wellspring. I maintain my painting and writing with great purpose, joy, and love.

Eli is sprouting like a weed. He is lanky and fine boned with a laser-tuned mind and graceful athleticism that serve him with stunning success. Sarah is all grown up now. She's off to college, studying hard to be a physician. They are treasures, these two, and their father and I have found a respectable modicum of parental cooperation. It is important to both of us that we raise the children well, so we hold true to our promises, providing loving security and structure.

Hunter had a horrid time in the year after Blue passed, but he has done a remarkable job at healing, himself. His dear daughter is gone forever, but their soul connection remains strong. He and I are bonded now in ways it takes a lifetime for others to achieve. I'm deeply grateful that, in spite of all that we've endured together, a sweet closeness and love between us still cocoons us in peace and safety.

Sadly, we lost my father in the aftermath of a massive stroke and buried him exactly ten years to the day that I became stricken with Lyme disease. My family tended lovingly to Dad in the ten days that it took for him to pass over. We sang and read, played Tommy Dorsey tapes to him, and opened all the windows to let in the June sunshine. As George's final hour approached, my family members, Hunter, and I gathered around him, our hearts ravaged and raw. At 3:30 p.m., after a still morning, a sudden, powerful southerly wind blew up the Hudson River just as Dad took his final breath, setting the leaves on the giant oak outside his riverview window into a dancing flurry. Simultaneously, from below, a long, steady whistle sounded on the northbound train. It was then that I knew that this wise and majestic man had set forth on his next great voyage. Another door closed in my life. But, as he would say to me in Greek, "A window opens." For me, in those luminous moments, time stood still.

I must say that I adore my house and neighborhood. It's terrific here, simple and sunny, welcoming and solid. The long solitude I endured through years of illness has been replaced by new friends, enlivened dinner parties, and backyard blueberry feasts, our yard rimmed with eighty-year-old heirloom bushes.

Lucky is king of the hill, sprawling out under the broad sugar maple on the front lawn for hours on end, surveying the environs and keeping watch over us, his happy corgi grin conveying supreme pleasure and faithful devotion. Happiness courses within all our veins.

This past winter, Hunter winterized the three-season sunporch for me, dropping the ceiling, installing insulation and radiant heaters, so I could have some studio space and a desk for writing. One summer's eve, as I sit here correcting a proof, the late-day sun streaks onto my shoulders, lighting up a nearby half-completed canvas in a butterscotch hue. I glance to my left, catching the view of the rosy sky and plump cumulus clouds. The new picture window Hunter had installed is rimmed with abundant greenery, rhododendrons, and spruce fingering the edges. It's lovely and peaceful out here, slightly removed from the household fray, surrounded by glass and light on three sides. As I stand, I catch a glimpse of a solitary mountain peak in the distance. Suddenly, a memory jolts through my mind:

This is the work space scene I conjured up at Stillpoint, over two years ago in Florida, when Meredith was helping us formulate our life's purpose and work in the world!

It strikes me yet again with absolute clarity that my intuitive training really is valid. *I guess we really can see into the future—or create our own—by seeding our visual and energetic intentions.*

I've learned so much in these few short years and I continue to grow in so many ways. In the course of this healing journey, patience and, ultimately, faith became the foundation on which I built my life's new structure. Yet there is always more to master. I look back a mere few years and see all that I held, believing it to be good and right. It was merely one form of reality, the culmination of what I had accrued over time according to society's standards of success. The jettisoning was hard, but necessary. The illness forced me to change.

Standing on a verdant plateau, I look back over the years from the high peak of experience and see a pathway covered in shattered glass. But there is a grand arcing rainbow stretching above it all. This is good.

I'm not proud of the broken marriages, the children with dueling households, or my years of fractured health. I wish I could've lived it all more elegantly. My life is not perfect. I do not have the luxuries many others claim at mid-age. I'm still juggling the elements of a more youthful age: minimal money, no steady job, child rearing still in full gear at age fifty-three. And I'm no longer a heroine. Instead I'm strong now in new ways, more steady and enduring.

I have ventured into the wilds of self and discovered both a mighty spirit within and an angel of mercy on my shoulder who would not let me give up. Many people and fortuitous circumstances bolstered me during this journey. I am deeply grateful, always.

In the meantime, I like the view from up here. It's peaceful, broad, and spectral. My vision is vast, my new perspective changing everything. I move to the edge, this time unafraid. Standing on a precipice, looking over the lustrous valley to the horizon, I see where I can fly to. How exciting! Out of the woods, trenches, and mires, I ease out my eagle's wings. They're achy from little use, but still familiar—broad and agile. On tiptoes I stretch up high, feeling the air around me, tasting the light and scents. Smiling, I scan around me. With a gentle push-off, I'm airborne, soaring out over the edge, catching the thermal updrafts. Alight and free, I'm flying out, up, and into the beyond. The world is mine. Just as my father told me as a very small child: I'm free and able to achieve anything!

I don't know exactly what awaits me, but now, soaring high with my inborn gifts of inner vision attuned, I have faith that I will meet it with grace.

May my story bring hope and help to those of you who need it. Healing is a journey of the deepest order. It comes from within. By opening your heart to its whispering, the answers will come. You will be set free. May each and every one of you be graced with the power of love. It is eternal. We are all eternal. This I know.

PART TWO

Lyme Disease— The Nuts and Bolts

In the fullness of time, the mainstream handling of chronic Lyme disease will be viewed as one of the most shameful episodes in the history of medicine because elements of academic medicine, elements of government, and virtually the entire insurance industry have colluded to deny a disease.

This has resulted in needless suffering of many individuals who deteriorate and sometimes die for lack of timely application of treatment or denial of treatment beyond some arbitrary duration.

—Kenneth Liegner, MD, address on Lyme disease at IOM meeting

Lyme disease leaves a person more sensitive, even after being healed. A more highly developed intuition and a more sensitive reaction to the environment are claimed to be part of a post–Lyme syndrome. They tend to cherish quiet meditation and a natural environment. Who knows? Maybe that is what the Borrelia entity is supposed to do. Maybe it is a way of Gaia (Mother Earth) to help people of today become more sensitive and responsive to the real world of nature.

—Wolf D. Storl, *Healing Lyme Disease Naturally*

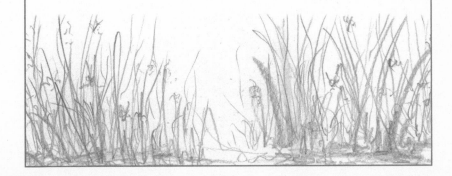

Signs and Symptoms

Lyme disease is a bacterial infection caused by an organism known as *Borrelia burgdorferi*. There are also variant Lyme tick-borne co-infections caused by similar microbes, *Ehrlichia*, *Babesia*, *Bartonella*, and mycoplasmas. These microorganisms and many other strains related to Lyme disease all cause a similar set of symptoms with some minor yet detectable characteristics differentiating them. *Borrelia* is classified as spirochete, or corkscrew bacteria, which is in the same family as syphilis, yet Lyme is considered to be stronger and more virulent. Like syphilis, Lyme initially starts with seemingly mild, acute symptomology, but over time, if untreated, it can cause devastating effects to the central nervous system, heart, kidneys, and endocrine, skeletal, and immune systems, with sometimes permanent repercussions. This panoply of systemic symptoms mimics many autoimmune-style disorders.

One of my most important messages to readers is that early diagnosis and detection of Lyme disease is critical. The sooner this bacterium is arrested, the more hopeful the prognosis is for a complete recovery. Do not hesitate to seek professional testing if you are at all suspicious you may have been infected by the bacteria. I can't stress this enough!

The bacterium is spread by a blood transfer. It's most commonly transmitted by the bite of a very tiny insect, the deer tick. These ticks are the size of a pinhead or small freckle. It has been commonly assumed that the tiny deer tick (*Ixodes scapularis*) is the only variety infected with *Borrelia burgdorferi* bacteria. This is incorrect. All species in the USA, Europe, Canada, Australia, Africa, Asia, and South America *can* be infected with Lyme disease (bb) and an assortment of co-infections. The lone star tick is particularly aggressive and quick to latch on to a host, often in less than one hour's time.

These co-infections are very tricky to diagnose properly via lab testing, still! A PCR test can sometimes confirm the organisms' presence. A clinical diagnosis is obtained via signs and symptoms collated by a Lyme disease specialist practitioner, most thoroughly trained beyond traditional medical, chiropractic, or naturopathic school, but also by the International Lyme and Associated Diseases Society (ILADS) or Tick-Borne Disease Alliance (TBDA). If your practitioner claims you do not test positive for Lyme disease and he or she is not ILADS or TBDA trained, seeking a second opinion is prudent.

Sexual relations may possibly transmit a form of the disease, noted in a January 2014 study including Dr. Ralph Stricker and Dr. Eva Sapi. Pregnant mothers may transfer the bacteria to their baby, as Lyme bacteria are capable of passing to the fetus through the placenta, as well as in breast milk in approximately 33 percent of mothers. Interestingly, however, some infected mothers do not spread the actual bacteria to the fetus, but the baby can be affected by central nervous system issues, ADHD, food allergies, autism, Tourette's syndrome, OCD, or other syndromes. The miasmatic influence from the mother instead sets up a host of sensitivities, allergies, or imbalances in the offspring. The term used referring to this syndrome is PANS: Peripheral Autonomic Nervous System.

Sharing food, drinks, or eating utensils, or shaking someone's hand has not been proved to transmit Lyme disease. It's potentially contagious through mucous membranes and saliva, but this is not confirmed. Our blood banks are contaminated and need screening. You can't catch it from your pets through natural contact, such as by grooming or caring for them. You can, however, get bitten by a tick carrying Lyme that is on their body and moves to yours. Sleeping with pets is discouraged. Washing their bedding and dousing them with repellent such as Vectra is wise.

Lyme disease is a rampant epidemic in the twenty-first century. Over thirty thousand diagnosed cases are reported annually to the CDC. In August 2013 the CDC announced actually over three hundred thousand people are infected yearly, yet these cases are not actually diagnosed or treated in acute onset form. Many authorities project that over one million cases are contracted annually in the USA. Lyme is now the most rampant infectious disease in the United States, four times ahead of HIV. In my own county in New Hampshire, it's been increasing at a rate of over 100 percent per year over the last five years, with over 75 to 90 percent of deer ticks infected with Lyme bacteria in certain counties. The eastern seaboard is under particularly fierce assault and the southern states are undereducated on the matter. Cases are multiplying in large numbers in the Ohio River Valley, across the Midwest, and along the West Coast as a wide variety of ticks now carry the disease. Mild winters do not kill them off. Eighty-nine countries of the world now report Lyme disease. Ticks themselves carry an array of other infectious illnesses such as Rocky Mountain spotted fever, various relapsing fevers, and viruses. Ticks are miniature cesspools. Essentially they transfer what they are carrying from a former host into you during their feeding cycle.

Low-lying woodland areas, beach grass, open meadows abutting forests, low shrubs, and ground covers like pachysandra are all favorable environments for ticks to inhabit. Ticks typically find a small animal, such as a rabbit, squirrel, raccoon, dog, or deer to live on as their host. They rest on leaves and grasses, about thigh-high, climbing aboard a warm-blooded animal (including humans) as they brush by. The tick crawls on the body, looking for soft, delicate skin as its entry point. They often gravitate to the nape of the neck, the armpits, and the groin. They will bite the host and attach, often lodging themselves for hours or days, as they engorge on blood. Many times the tick will never completely lodge itself in its host, but merely just crawl about. It must lodge itself in order to transfer the bacteria. Some suggest the tick must be embedded for over twenty-four hours for the blood transfer, but data does not support this well-intended reassuring conclusion. It all depends on where the tick is in its feeding cycle when it adheres to you.

Spring is a particularly elevated time for tick numbers, as this is when their eggs hatch, releasing almost translucent nymphs, which are particularly hard to see. After a rain, their population can be heavier, too. Autumn brings another round of infestation.

The most telltale sign of a new Lyme infection is the "bull's-eye" rash or bite from the tick. A red dot in the center, with an outer red circle, is the classic early warning sign. This target-shaped rash may be as small as a dime or as large as a softball. Sometimes it's a pale pink color, other times it's a vermillion red, even inflamed to a swollen, sore, black-and-blue degree. Sometimes people show just a welt. This "erythema migrans" rash is a 100 percent confirmation that you have been infected by *Borrelia burgdorferi* when a tick accompanies it.

Many people never notice such a bite. Only approximately 50 percent show the target rash. I did not. But then again, I lived deep in the woods and we were always covered with blackfly and mosquito bites, resembling a connect-the-dot diagram. A small bull's-eye could also be in a not-so-visible place, such as your back or scalp. If you think a red welt or bite could be a common spider bite—also sometimes a red dot encircled with a red ring—again, please get it examined. With Lyme disease escalating so rapidly and its consequences being so dire, it's not worth brushing off such a bite as insignificant. Men, please note: you're not being a wimp if you have an insect bite examined!

Aside from the initial bull's-eye rash, other early symptoms of a Lyme infection can include an aching, flu-like feeling, often noted in the limbs, back, and neck. Mild chills or nausea may accompany these pains. Occasionally, individuals exhibit a frank swelling or pronounced pain in their joints (the knee being the most common). A slight fever, rarely over 100 degrees, is not atypical. Headaches, often severe, are the second most common symptom alongside the flu-like feeling. Dizziness, sore throat, fatigue, and swollen glands may all manifest as well. Depression is not atypical.

As was plainly evident in my case, any constellation of the mentioned symptomology tends to linger beyond a few days without blossoming into the customary respiratory or gastrointestinal pathway of influenza. The heavy mucus production, sinus drainage, and cough of the flu usually do not occur. This is a very significant feature to note. If you're feeling unwell and flu-ish, but not progressing into the natural route of sinus and cough, think Lyme. What later sets in is the heavy malaise and pronounced fatigue, often accompanied by a "cottony head" sensation and mental dullness. Some cases occasionally bloom into a pronounced influenza state, whereby one discounts the notion of Lyme at all. Individuals with very strong immune systems may get these flu-like symptoms for only a few days, to relapse again weeks or even months later.

Please note that children may not get all the mentioned symptoms. Instead they most commonly manifest achiness and headaches, and maybe the bull's-eye bite. Because children so frequently experience mild fevers, sore throats, and tiredness associated with a touch of some passing viral infection going through their school or day care, we tend just to ride out their discomforts for a few days or a week, assuming it will all pass as their active immune systems capably arrest the microbe invasion. Most often this mind-set is adequate and the child ably recovers from common viruses.

If your child complains of headaches, is unfocused in school, is showing anxiety or restlessness, has a knee or other joint that hurts, or just doesn't seem to have his or her usual energy a few weeks after a seemingly mild cold or flu-like episode, again I encourage you to have him or her tested for Lyme disease. Children, teens, and very healthy adults often are misdiagnosed regarding early Lyme infections, especially if they didn't exhibit the bull's-eye rash or you didn't find a tick on their body. Their immune systems are very active and strong, working aggressively to tamp down the *Borrelia* right away. Emotional woes, ADD, anger attacks, and sleep disorders are common even in healthy youngsters and teens. Headaches, depression, OCD, anxiety, malaise, and GI issues are very common in kids, and so may not raise suspicion. The result is early, undiagnosed signs of Lyme, then a quieter waiting period, with malingering symptoms sometimes resurfacing weeks or months later, whereby no one, doctor or patient, makes the correlation to the initial infection. This scenario is where most chronic Lyme cases have gone awry. They were not diagnosed in the office or via accurate laboratory testing and clinical assessment up front, setting up the individual for repeated suspicious outbreaks, eventually morphing into the mysterious and vague status of chronic Lyme disease, sometimes with serious neurological or cardiac consequences. A lifetime of suffering can ensue.

Many physicians aren't willing to acknowledge the concept of chronic Lyme disease, as the IDSA has not gotten completely on board with this condition, still claiming Lyme disease is only an acute illness of a limited duration, and calling lingering symptoms "Post-Lyme Syndrome." Yet chronic Lyme disease is a very evasive condition, defying a clear black-and-white set of diagnostic keynotes. It may attack one or more primary systems of the body, consequently creating a broad variety of symptoms variant from case to case. The endocrine system gets particularly skewed.

Dr. Worthington was correct to say that I got off easy with my debilitating case of Lyme disease. I have met others whose neurological systems have been attacked, resulting in Parkinson's, various types of palsy, MS, ALS, neuropathy, Crohn's, bipolar disorder, obsessive-compulsive disorder, and hallucinations. I've counseled individuals who have heart troubles, such as pericarditis, or valve problems from the Lyme bacteria. A friend's child had ocular Lyme and was blind until treated. Many people are hospitalized from Lyme disease, especially when the immune system becomes so overburdened that secondary infections, like pneumonia, Epstein-Barr virus, Bell's palsy, MS, or ME, hit. Water on the knee, rheumatoid arthritis, stiff necks, fibromyalgia, migraines, CFS, and lupus are common signs of a chronic case of Lyme and errant testing.

Being that the musculoskeletal system, immune/lymphatic system, gastrointestinal system, heart/circulation system, neurological system, and skin each can be attacked, again variant from case to case, a panoply of sometimes perplexing symptoms can evade a clear-cut diagnosis. A clinical diagnosis is made by a symptom picture, backed up with new state-of-the-art laboratory testing that identifies DNA fragments of Lyme bacteria and specific proteins more closely. With limited funds, a few valiant research docs are diligently working to crack the code.

One of my greatest concerns regarding the millions of people with progressed Lyme disease cases is for the broken spirits that can result from this debilitating, ruinous illness. A being can handle only so much. Lyme takes the physical, mental, and emotional stuffing out of so many people and their caregivers. Tending to the broken spirit is just as critical as mending a broken body. This rampaging epidemic has shown us its very ugly face. Hundreds of thousands of people are suffering at so many levels because of it. My plea is that we must find resources to tend to those afflicted. Reach out to organizations such as ILADS, TBDA, LRA,

Lymedisease.org, and Lyme-MS-Pathology.com to find studies going on, and donate your blood or financial support.

Note: Lyme disease is technically caused by the bacteria *Borrelia burgdorferi*. The similar co-infections are bacterial, parasitic, or mycoplasmic. For brevity's sake, the rest of the Nuts and Bolts section will refer to Lyme disease as a bacteria.

Please see www.OutoftheWoodsBook.com for a complete reference list.

Lyme Disease Symptom Questionnaire Checklist Of Symptomology

Lyme disease can present with a broad array of symptomology. More than one system of the body may be affected. The format below clusters complaints referable to specific organ systems. If you note ten or more symptoms, especially moderate or severe, seeking professional help and testing is strongly encouraged.

Have you had any of the following? *refers to symptoms most unique to Lyme disease.

Tick bite	Y	N		Bull's-eye rash (red circle with dot in center)	Y	N
Spotted rash over large area	Y	N		Linear, red streaks	Y	N

SYMPTOM OR SIGN	CURRENT SEVERITY			
	NONE	MILD	MODERATE	SEVERE
Flu-like symptoms (fever, chills, cough, aching)				
Headache/stiff neck				
Meningitis				
General malaise				
Apathy and mental dullness				

Persistent swollen glands				
Sore throat				
Fevers				
Sore soles, especially in the a.m.				
* Joint pain				
Fingers, toes				
Ankles, wrists				
Knees, elbows				
Hips, shoulders				
Joint swelling				
Fingers, toes				
Ankles, wrists				
Knees, elbows				
Hips, shoulders				
Unexplained back pain or hip pain, lying on side produces hip pain				

Stiffness of the joints or back				
Muscle pain or cramps				
Obvious muscle weakness, legs feel unable to support, rising from seat laborious and painful				
Twitching or paralysis of the face or other muscles				
Tremors and/or jittery feeling				
Seizures				
Headache, including migraine				
Light sensitivity				
Sound sensitivity				
Vision: double, blurry, floaters, dry eyes				
Ear pain, prolonged or repeated episodes				

Hearing: buzzing, ringing, decreased hearing			
Increased motion sickness, vertigo, spinning			
Off balance, "tippy" feeling			
Tingling, numbness, burning, or stabbing sensations, shooting pains, skin hypersensitivity – worse on left side			
Facial paralysis – Bell's palsy			
Dental pain			
* Neck creaks and cracks, stiffness, neck pain			
* Fatigue, tired, poor stamina, exhaustion, collapse			
* Insomnia, fractionated sleep, early awakening			

Excessive nighttime sleep				
Napping during the day				
Unexplained weight gain				
Unexplained weight loss				
Unexplained hair loss				
Pain in genital area				
Unexplained menstrual irregularity				
Unexplained milk production, breast pain				
Irritable bladder or bladder dysfunction, repeated UTIs (urinary tract infections)				
Erectile dysfunction				
Loss of libido				

Queasy stomach or nausea			
Heartburn, stomach pain			
Constipation			
Diarrhea			
Low abdominal pain, cramps			
Heart murmur or valve prolapse			
Heart palpitations or skips, atrial fibrillation			
"Heart block" on EKG			
Chest wall pain or sore ribs, clutching sensation in ribs/ chest			
Head congestion			
Breathlessness, "air hunger," unexplained chronic cough			
Night sweats			

Exaggerated symptoms or worse hangover from alcohol				
* Symptom flares every four weeks				
Gray skin pallor				
Unexplained skin rash or eruption				
Elevated white blood count				
Elevated lymphocyte count				
Persistent yeast/ fungal infections				
Confusion, difficulty thinking				
Difficulty with concentration, reading, problem absorbing new information, brain fog				
Word search, name block				

Forgetfulness, poor short-term memory, poor attention				
Disorientation: getting lost, going to wrong places				
Speech errors: wrong word, misspeaking				
Mood swings, irritability, depression, suicidal feelings				
Anxiety, panic attacks, overreaction to news, even minor events				
Psychosis (hallucinations, delusions, paranoia, bipolar)				

Prevention

Being aware of Lyme disease and co-infection symptoms is a must for all of us these days, just as it used to be important to watch for polio symptoms. We can no longer be relaxed about this exploding epidemic, with irregular weather patterns inducing rampant tick reproduction and expanding habitats for them to thrive in.

As a child in Vermont in the 1970s I never saw a tick, even when camping outdoors for weeks on end. The winters were fierce in northern New England, Minnesota, and Wisconsin, killing ticks off with January cold stretches of -20° F for many frigid weeks in a row. Winter weather like that is rare these days, and nonexistent in lower latitudes. As a result, Lyme-infected ticks are commonly found in bucolic Vermont, in the meandering lakes of Wisconsin, throughout Canada, and are here to stay in pandemic numbers in the southern climes.

A shockingly sad story relayed to me by a lovely woman in Tennessee summed up the naivete of many medical professionals in the South.

June 2012:

"Katina, my husband was out clearing brush on our property and when he came in I plucked fifteen ticks off of him. Five had these big red bull's-eye rings," she said, her eyes wide with alarm.

"I told him, 'Honey, I think you've got Lyme disease. We'd better see the doctor.'" Nodding yes in apt concurrence, my heart lurched when she continued.

"Our doctor examined my husband, didn't even take a blood test, and said to us, 'Oh that's not Lyme disease, we don't have that illness down here. It is only found on Cape Cod. Those are spider bites. Take some Benadryl.'"

"He sent us home and my husband has been so sick for over a solid year now. He has crippling migraines, swollen knees, horrid back pains, and sleeps nonstop. He had to quit his job. I don't know what to do."

Another life maimed by misinformation, lack of medical training, and lax IDSA reaction to this epidemic. I sent them to a top-notch Lyme-literate MD out of state and this man is on over a year of treatments and thankfully is improving.

The stories I've heard in twenty-four months on the road are endless and all too similar. We *must* practice prevention and pay attention to *all* suspicious symptoms. You have control over prevention. Key steps are as follows.

We love the beaches, the woods, and our gardens and golf courses. When returning from gardening, hiking, horseback riding—any outdoor quests—strip off all clothes in your foyer, mudroom, laundry room, or garage, and put them immediately in the dryer on the hottest heat setting for thirty minutes. High heat will kill ticks (which is why there are fewer in the desert Southwest).

Other prevention measures or tick deterrents are to keep your yards or socializing areas wide open to the sun and the grass closely shorn. Have *no* loose shrubbery, pachysandra, creeping myrtle, swaying grasses, or bird feeders near your house or patio. Ticks prefer damp, darker areas. Woodpiles, fern beds, and autumn leaf piles are danger zones. Keep woodpiles out of your garage or mudroom.

Sadly, birds are enormous threats to our safety. As lovely as these colorful, pretty creatures are, they are "tick taxis," transporting millions of infected *Ixodes* on their migratory flyways. A large Canada goose can carry over one thousand, a tiny warbler dozens. Beautiful California, Florida, Paraguay, Canada, and Norway are now ransacked with tickborne diseases, as birds have brought infected ticks everywhere en route!

Keep bird feeders far from your social space, at the distant perimeters of your property, as a tick can readily drop off and creep aboard your pet, your child, or even you.

Ticks will not crawl on pebbles, gravel, flagstone, or brick as a rule of thumb. Many folks create nice stone patio areas for dining and sunning or around a pool. Keep swing sets and sandboxes away from woodland edges, and keep them in the sun, laying a terrain of gravel in a three-foot-perimeter fashion to deter ticks from crawling near your children.

It is very sad for "woodland spirit" me to admit that free rambles in the open meadows and tree climbing in forest glades are now risky for youngsters. Educate them and use repellents, please.

Encourage your school systems, recreation departments, sports teams, outing clubs, garden clubs, and state park systems to provide seasonal Lyme disease education and post warning signs.

Always check your limbs and clothing when coming back from a walk. Where I live we do daily tick checks when coming in from outdoors and scan our bodies, feeling behind ears, in the hair, and along our limbs at bedtime. It's wise to check your family pets regularly, too. Of course, spraying with insect repellent before going into the woods, meadows, and beach dunes is wise and strongly recommended as a deterrent. DEET does not always deter ticks. A repellent such as Repel, containing permethrin (derived from chrysanthemum), is more effective. Natural offerings made from lemon balm, eucalyptus, and rose geranium are safe on children and on the skin. Long sleeves, pant legs, and socks help, too. Please check your young children daily and teach the older ones to examine themselves nightly, just as you routinely brush your teeth. A clothing line called Insect Shield is doused in permethrin and is good for seventy washings.

Consider having your pets vaccinated against Lyme disease. LymeVax has been thoroughly studied and implemented successfully with millions of doses in the past decade. You can also use tick/flea baths and sprays to prevent the insects from biting your pets. Frontline and Vectra are known to be effective, animal-friendly repellents. The black-legged tick, American dog tick, lone star tick, western black-legged tick, and Pacific Coast tick—all Lyme carriers—can be deterred this way. Brush your pets outside daily and check for ticks.

We have some other new products available to help with prevention measures. There's a simple, handy, unique item called "Tick Tubes," made by a company called Damminix. Resembling the inner cardboard of a paper-towel roll, these "Tubes" are stuffed with permethrin-doused cotton. You place them in assorted locations around your property where rodents may venture—a woodpile, a stone wall, an attic, a garage, a tree crook, etc.

Chipmunks, mice, or squirrels will gather some of this cotton batting to feather their nests, in turn killing off ticks on their own bodies and offspring, reducing numbers on your property. A farmer in Massachusetts relayed to me that in the summer of 2011 she was pulling ten to fifteen ticks per day off her cats and dogs, and more from her horses. Using "Tick Tubes" in 2012, she found a mere one or two per week on the horses, and often none on the dogs and cats! Plant nurseries or online sources stock this item.

Pest control companies can spray your yards with permethrin or cedar oil to keep ticks away. Many reputable outfits abound in the USA. See the resource section in the appendix. If you live in a high-density tick area, like the Carolinas, Kansas, the Northeast, or the Pacific Northwest, you may want to consider routine spraying.

We do not have a human Lyme vaccine. In the 1980s one was introduced and it backfired, giving people active Lyme disease, and many still have persistent symptoms. They pulled the vaccine from the market. Remember, *Borrelia b.* is related to syphilis. We do not have a syphilis vaccine either.

"Insider" talk rumors a newer Lyme vaccine is to be introduced. Lyme-literate physicians and researchers are quite leery about this product, however, since all the actual physiological responses involved in Lyme disease's multiplex systemic relays are still not patently understood. Are there genetic predispositions to this infection going "wild" in some people, such as an autoimmune trigger, genome flaws in certain people, liver enzyme inadequacies in others, mitochondria dysfunction, or even brain neurotransmitter sensitivities? Until these key-pins and further physiology are clearly established, a new Lyme vaccine could be another "setup" for many unsuspecting individuals to get quite ill. Awareness and practicing prevention are still the safest and wisest measures, just as we do with HIV.

A final note on the prevention topic: get your state government involved in the Lyme disease issue. New York, Massachusetts, Connecticut, and Virginia have been fiercely working with their state legislators to get Lyme disease bills passed of assorted measures.

Monte Skall and Susan Green got Virginia House Bill 1933 passed, establishing that a negative Lyme disease test result does not mean that your doctor can rule out Lyme disease as your diagnosis. Tune in to LymeLightRadio.com archived show September 25, 2013, to learn more on how you can work for similar legislation in your state. Thank you, Ms. Green and NatCapLyme founder, Ms. Skall.

Staci Grodin, president of Tick-Borne Disease Alliance, in a LymeLightRadio.com December 18, 2013 interview explains how to help get a national Lyme disease bill passed in Washington, DC, with your personal assistance.

Trish McCleary of S.L.A.M. (Sturbridge Lyme Awareness of Massachusetts) and Duvall Patrick have declared May as Lyme Disease Awareness Month, now an international campaign, and are working on Lyme Bill No. H989 for insurance company coverage beyond sixty days in Massachusetts.

Helping each state or country establish Lyme disease medical, insurance company, and legal precedence is a critical step in defining this surging epidemic and prompting help for everyone's vulnerability. Visit TBDAlliance.org to learn more.

Meanwhile, practicing prevention and awareness measures in your personal lifestyle is essential! The situation with ticks now being severely infected and infested is alarming in many instances. Our loggers, farmers, and park rangers are very vulnerable, and so is anyone with a yard, on a hike, on a golf course, or near the woods. Be alert, be proactive, and educate your family, friends, neighbors, and physicians!

If you do find a tick embedded in your body, carefully and slowly remove it with tweezers. Contact IGeneX Labs or Mainelyticks.com to mail the tick in for testing, to see what it is infected with. If treatment is required, the sooner you start aggressive antibiotic therapy for an acute infection, the better the odds are for a quick recovery.

Laboratory Testing

The *Borrelia*, *Ehrlichia*, *Bartonella*, and *Babesia* organisms of Lyme disease are not always successfully identified in the bloodstream of an individual or pet via various aspects of laboratory testing. The trick is using the correct test and lab to identify the organism's presence. Even then, accuracy is not 100 percent; we do not yet have one definitive Lyme disease diagnostic test. Lyme disease can be elusive. The symptoms and the cycles of "active" versus "dormant" outbreaks make it difficult and frustrating to identify the bacteria's presence. Often, a person knows he or she is sick, yet a physician, hospital, or laboratory will tell that person time and again that he or she is fine. Meanwhile, the Lyme is silently embedding itself further and further into the person's tissues and organs. Others end up with a suspicious lupus, ALS, MS, or rheumatoid arthritis diagnosis, while thousands are lumped into a fibromyalgia or chronic fatigue syndrome misdiagnosis.

My second strongest message to readers who are suspicious that they may have Lyme disease is to insist that your doctor use one of the more sensitive labs (IGeneX, Clongen, Neuroscience) and their specific tests in order to obtain an accurate result. The vast majority of doctors not specializing in treating Lyme disease have relied on the common ELISA (enzyme-linked immunosorbent assay) Lyme test or the commercial lab Western blot Lyme test at a local or regional facility, for the past decade or more, as the sole method of identifying the Lyme bacteria in the bloodstream. These two tests are extremely inaccurate and faulty, with up to a 70 percent false-negative error rate.

One reason for this statistic is that the ELISA and Western blot Lyme panels ordered from most local hospitals and labs are typically not sensitive enough to detect the presence of the Lyme bacteria unless it happens to be exactly during the few-weeks window these tests can zero in on.

The newest, most specific and sensitive tests are major assets in battling chronic Lyme by making a more accurate diagnosis feasible. The CDC and ISDA currently do not recognize the chronicity of Lyme bacteria's presence, making it difficult for physicians to diagnose or treat when all they receive is a negative test result on a patient with the antibody, ELISA, or Western blot tests. At the International Conference on Lyme Borreliosis and Other Tick-Borne Diseases in Boston 2013, the concept of "Post–Lyme Syndrome" was acknowledged by the IDSA. This is not a statement agreeing that Lyme disease can take a "chronic form," mimicking MS, ALS, or CFS. Rather, their words suggest the recommended fourteen to thirty days of antibiotic therapy for acute Lyme disease "may" kill the *Borrelia*, but something else is at play when patients end up with chronic symptoms; that is, autoimmune illness and inflammation cascades are triggered.

There is much more to unearth surrounding *Borrelia* and the very common co-infections a person suffers with. Dr. Richard Horowitz, past president of ILADEF, author of *Why Can't I Get Better? Solving the Mystery of Lyme and Chronic Disease*, has treated over twelve thousand Lyme disease patients. He states that the co-infections are a significant leader in the persistent, debilitated cases. Accurate diagnostic testing is of extremely high precedence. Currently, Lyme-literate practitioners make a clinical diagnosis and feel reassured when more than one lab test gives them positive confirmation.

Dr. Ahmed Kilani of Clongen Labs has devoted much time and research to Lyme disease. He confirms that when testing for *Borrelia burgdorferi* we are looking for merely one strain of that organism, and there are many strains of the bacteria and the co-infections.

His statistics cite:
* 117 total organism strains

- 32 *Borrelia* (up to 300 known internationally)
- 29 *Bartonella*
- 6 *Babesia*
- 6 *Anaplasma*
- 12 *Ehrlichia*
- 23 *Rickettsia*

And this does not include the viruses, mycoplasmas, and Rocky Mountain spotted fever, or other organisms, such as FL1953 protozoa (Fry Labs), that a tick may carry. Other studies suggest three hundred worldwide *Borrelia* strains. No wonder upward of one million people are infected annually with tick-borne diseases and a mere fraction are properly diagnosed.

Every six months or so a clearer lens into the mechanisms of the shape-shifting *Borrelia* spirochete is illuminated. Researchers and laboratories are earnestly attempting to find an infallible testing method to diagnose *Borrelia's* presence, both immediately upon infection (in the example of a tick bite), and the more persistent cases.

There are tests worth speaking to your practitioner about. Both IGeneX and Clongen Labs have much more sensitive Western blot antibody tests, PCR, immune modulator tests, and co-infection tests than commercial labs. The bands that show up positive on the Western blot test that help a practitioner confirm a *Borrelia* infection are numbers 23, 31, 34, 39, and 83 to 93.

Additionally, an experienced, Lyme-savvy practitioner will want to see another positive confirmation elsewhere, such as on a CD 57 test (LabCorp). The lower the number on this test, the more aggressively your immune system is working to fight off an infection (Lyme, EBV, HIV all included, however).

DNA fragments of *Borrelia* found in the urine is another confirmation. IGeneX's urine etiope test is one version, and Ceres's Nanotrap test, being put through rigid clinical trials at George Mason University, may be a breakthrough moment in Lyme disease diagnostics. This test works on examining antigens in the urine. Antigens are the first reactors to a microbial infection, versus the later-forming antibodies. This Nanotrap test is currently the most clearly promising indicative tool for an early, acute infection.

The other test of growing success is Neuroscience Labs' iSpot Lyme™ test. This test relies on the activation of the patient's effector T cells (immune response). It utilizes four antigens instead of two and detects the signature proteins called cytokines. The results are qualified as a function of the increase in the levels of interferon gamma. iSpot Lyme™ is a highly reliable and accurate test, with an 84 percent sensitivity rate and specificity of 94 percent. Many doctors are turning to this method now.

Additionally, Neuroscience offers an ELISPOT, another antigen test, which confirms *Borrelia* presence in many seronegative Western blot or ELISA cases.

Still in question are the blood culture tests being performed. A patient's blood sample is allowed to culture on specific "agars" for two to twelve weeks, noting if *Borrelia* or certain co-infections grow, akin to a urinary tract infection culture test. At first the outlook was promising. But now, two years later, the process is questionable, as there is a preponderance of "positive" test results, suggesting that the test may produce a false positive too often.

Working with a Lyme-literate practitioner is a wise choice if an autoimmune illness diagnosis is given to you. Lyme can induce a positive ANA lupus test, or RA factor test for rheumatoid arthritis, and MS is very often confused as Lyme disease. A symptom questionnaire is included starting on page 260.

The average MD does not know about these specific tests or the specialty labs focusing on Lyme. Insist that these facilities be used or find a Lyme-literate physician who is savvy about this important subject. More insurance companies, including Medicare, now reimburse for some of the tests, which is a real boon. Please explore these labs. They are turning lives around in thousands of instances. Read their web pages for the specifics on new case tests and those for chronic, older cases, as they differ. Your practitioner can interface with these labs on technical questions. Once a diagnosis is achieved, proper treatment can begin. Diligence, patience, and persistence are all important.

Treatment Options

Author's Healing Philosophy

As you realize by now, I am a classical homeopath who managed to recover from an advanced case of chronic neurological Lyme disease by the use of natural medicine treatments. Initially, it was a frustrating situation to be a "patient." I learned a great deal about myself, though—the powers of the body and spirit, as well as how and when both Western and alternative medicine practices come into play with chronic illness. Though there are volumes I could say about creating a healthier and more effective health-care system here in the United States, I will for now acknowledge that the USA is in dire need of a much more integrated medicine system. We are behind the times compared to Europe, Canada, and South America when it comes to utilizing complementary medicine alongside allopathic drugs. Treating the whole person, not just the disease, is crucial.

Lyme disease is a vastly more serious and involved illness than much of the health-care world realizes. Millions of people are gravely suffering and there is no simple, one-way route to getting well. Even Lyme specialists are still searching for answers. It appears at present that multiple modalities need to be incorporated to achieve a state of wellness in many chronic cases. Early acute cases can be swiftly and successfully cured with prompt aggressive antibiotic treatment for a minimum of six to twelve weeks as ILADS suggests. Older cases can be complex.

I believe this is the epidemic crisis of our era, one that asks us to join the two hands of health care: the diagnostic and pharmaceutical weaponry of allopathic medicine with the supportive therapeutics of natural medicine. Two hands working together are better than one. It seems the best recovery requires multiple approaches utilized in a harmonious blend, hopefully all under one roof in the years to come.

The pages ahead highlight some of the more available and effective methods to treat Lyme disease. Please seek professional medical guidance regarding your case. Lyme is a serious, complicated illness. It cannot be cured by self-help measures, but requires the expertise of a Lyme-literate health-care practitioner.

The overarching philosophy that I embraced, and have seen confirmed by the most progressive practitioners reaching most optimal results, involves four cornerstones:

1.   Open up the body's natural detoxification pathways first—liver, kidneys, lymphatics, and spleen—using natural products and therapies.
2.   Use metabolic profile analysis tests (e.g., Genova, ConVerge Labs) to assess where depletions lie and which systems are most damaged. Build in restorative nutritive supplements, herbs, homeopathics, and acupuncture for restoration.
3.   Address killing off all the "bugs" with antibiotics/pharmaceuticals, herbals, and Rife technology.
4.   Tend to the emotional and spiritual wounds chronic illness induces. A journey of personal transformation is happening. Spiritual healers, shamans, and ministers are vital helpers in this domain.

The author and this book do not attempt to treat Lyme disease, but instead offer information for investigative purposes as a means of suggesting healing options to explore. The author takes no responsibility for promising any cures to the reader, nor purports to know the right way to get well. Lyme disease necessitates an individual exam and an experienced health-care provider's clinical supervision. Seek help, please! And dig deep! You must embrace willpower, belief, faith, and fortitude. Build support networks into your life as needed.

Antibiotic Therapy

Antibiotic therapy is the fundamental tool conventional Western medicine has to offer regarding treatment of Lyme disease. It's a strong and effective tool when used appropriately with Lyme. In the early weeks of a new Lyme infection, six to twelve weeks of the tetracycline/doxycycline drug class can kill the fresh bacterial invasion immediately. This is the best and most promising time to employ antibiotics, killing the microbe before it has time to reproduce in the body.

If early identification of Lyme disease is not achieved and several months have lapsed, then four or more months of rotational antibiotic therapy is recommended as the current protocol. Because the Lyme bacteria replicate every four weeks, after three to four months of infestation several generations of microbes reside in one's bloodstream and tissues, necessitating multiple rounds of antibiotics. Plus, more microorganisms can be present, such as parasites, mycoplasmas, and viruses. Symptom nuances will help a doctor decide if you need antimalarials, antiparasitics, or antifungals, too.

Chronic cases of Lyme disease that have been going on for more than a year could require anywhere from four months to numerous years of antibiotic therapy, as the infection is extremely entrenched, existing now in three forms: spirochete bacteria, spherocyte, and cyst. Cysts are the so-called dormant phase of the disease cycle, whereby someone can actually be asymptomatic. Hence, the elusive, hide-and-seek quality of the disease, propagating mysterious episodes of malaise, confusion, headaches, pain, anxiety attacks, and diarrhea alternating with wellness.

Not all antibiotics kill the bacteria in the walled-off, hidden cyst stage. A class of pharmaceuticals in the 5-nitroimidazole/"Flagyl" family is often used, as well as those in the antiparasitic and antimalarial families. This is also the phase at which the Rife technology, certain herbals, and homeopathic remedies can do the work, too. When a hatch-out occurs, either spontaneously or when the system is stressed via seasonal climate change, a trauma or accident, surgery, or upsetting emotions, the next generational outbreak of bacteria needs to be killed off with another six weeks of pharmaceutical therapy. With this understanding, one can fathom how a ten-year-old case of Lyme disease may require two to three years of rotational pharmaceutical drug treatments, plus additional supportive modalities, as one moves in and out of the various phases of the bacterium's life cycle.

Early cases of Lyme usually respond to oral antibiotics. Chronic cases may necessitate IV use, being a more direct approach that also ransacks the GI tract less severely. Any long-term antibiotic use, though, will require good digestive flora boosting with probiotics and fermented foods such as kefir, sauerkraut, and yogurts.

There is some question regarding the amoxicillin class of antibiotics sometimes turned to in the early bacterial invasion stage, or cell-wall stage. It appears that this type of antibiotic will destroy the outer cell wall of the spirochete, but it leaves a morphing survival-oriented microbe in its place, which will then readily embed itself in the body's tissues and go into the propagating secondary, protein-synthesis stage. This is not a desirable situation. Some doctors refuse to use amoxicillin, as it sets up a situation of the Lyme actually self-propagating in a more aggressive form and making a more entrenched infection. The tetracycline and macrolide classes of antibiotics are preferable, as well as Rife technology and/or herbals if someone is not able to take the tetracycline antibiotics.

The tetracyclines can produce profound skin sun sensitivity, with horrid burns and rashes occurring. A well-versed Lyme physician is paramount regarding seasonal climates and antibiotic use. As a homeopath, I'm not experienced in antibiotic protocols. Much of my research and education from medical professionals I interviewed has alerted me to this information, however, making it seem necessary to point out—and critical in acute cases. Make sure to discuss this with your practitioner.

Chronic Lyme is a complex condition. Antibiotic use must be approached with the support of a Lyme-literate MD or ND who has strong experience with rotational drugs, as well as the ability to identify what stage the disease is in throughout the individual's treatment regimen. Adjunctive support of the alternative modalities and detoxification efforts can facilitate a more effective and timely course of treatment, offering people the best balance of healing efforts while reclaiming their lives from the trenches of this enormously debilitating disease.

Unfortunately, various state governments are trying to limit medical doctors' use of long-term antibiotic therapy by insinuating that the chronic form of Lyme disease is a fabricated illness. Legal and political wars are raging around this controversy. This book does not seek to explore these issues. Lyme websites and newspapers can present information on such matters.

Antibiotics Commonly Used with Lyme Disease and Co-Infections:

(Courtesy of Dr. Joseph Burrascano Jr., "Advanced Topics on Lyme Disease," 2005)

- doxycycline
- cefuroxime axetil
- erythromycin
- amoxicillin
- azithromycin
- clarithromycin
- telithromycin
- augmentin
- chloramphenicol
- metronidazole
- benzathine penicillin
- vancomycin (potential toxic limits)
- ampicillin

Babesia:
- mepron
- malarone
- azithromycin
- clarithromycin

Bartonella:
- levofloxacin
- rifampin
- cephalosporins
- azithromycin

Erlichia:
- doxycycline

See www.OutoftheWoodsBook.com for an up-to-date list of recommended MDs and other informational websites.

Complementary Medicine

Some readers may already be advocates of alternative or complementary medicine, having used disciplines like chiropractic or Reiki. Others may not have delved into this arena, instead relying on mainstream allopathic Western medicine for their doctoring needs. I will take a moment to mention the philosophy behind the holistic approaches of some of the more broad-reaching disciplines within the domain of complementary medicine, or natural medicine, as I like to refer to it.

Over the past decade, a segment of Western medically schooled, allopathic doctors have been broadening their scope from a solely pharmaceutical/surgery-based philosophy, and seeking additional post–medical school training to include complementary medicine protocols in their "toolbox" of practice skills. You will see terms such as "functional medicine" or "integrative medicine" on a physician's shingle or in a clinic's name. For clarification purposes, this newer bloom in American medicine means this type of physician may also use nutritional supplements, herbs, acupuncture, etc. in his or her practice. My personal hope is that this trend continues, as we need these two hands of medicine working together.

In the United States, the term "natural medicine" refers to healing disciplines that do not rely on drugs and surgery as their treatment protocols, but instead turn to methods based either on sources from the natural world or practices that may be centuries or even thousands of years old. Some of these practices were lost or abandoned in our Western approach to doctoring in the 1900s, as the fast-moving influx of pharmacology and the scientific emphasis in Western medicine came to dominate our American culture. The majority of the scientific and medical discoveries of the twentieth century have been incredible and lifesaving. In the massive forward advancement of scientific exploration in the United States, however, some of the gentler, more time-honored techniques of natural healing were ignored and actually frowned upon for many decades.

I can recall my chiropractor uncle needing to keep a low profile in his work space in the 1960s, for fear of AMA antagonism. Fortunately, the latter part of the twentieth century brought a shift of perspectives and attitudes about many of the more established natural healing methods, such as acupuncture and naturopathic medicine. Now, the United States is becoming more like Europe and South America, where an appropriate understanding and acceptance of the holistic disciplines is more respected. Perhaps the greatest stumbling block at this point in our health-care model is that scant amounts of money have been allocated, either federally or privately, to investigate scientifically just what makes some of these ancient and progressive natural healing modalities so successful, and how.

The main point to understand with the natural healing practices mentioned in this book is that they follow the holistic doctrines of aiming to treat the person in totality, not just the microcosm of his or her disease. Essentially, one's symptoms are not treated by drug modification routes, but the whole body is supported and balanced via the discipline's tools. Symptoms are looked at as signs and guides, and are not just squelched.

If you are new to holistic thinking, it may take a bit of mental readjustment to understand that we want to work with our bodies and emotions, not against them. We want to honor what our system is telling us via its symptomology and glean this information, taking it to our practitioner so he or she may find the correct remedy, supplements, acupuncture points, and so on that most effectively stimulate the innate healing abilities. The goal is to respect, care for, and applaud our body and psyche for their perseverance and note the magnificent efforts they maintain to keep us alive.

The chapters ahead outline the basics of the natural health-care approaches I integrated in my treatment of chronic Lyme disease. In my studies, readings, and interviews with others, time and again I found positive claims from those people who also turned to these modalities and used them in a thorough, durable fashion. Natural medicine does not provide quick fixes, but stable, longer-range results. If you recall my earlier statement, chronic Lyme disease cures are most solidly achieved with the use of integrative medicine. This means pharmaceutical treatments are integrated with the restorative therapeutic world of natural medicine. Rebuilding depletions and damage are essential.

These methods here worked for me, but they might not be the exact constellation that works for you. Lyme is so tricky and complicated in the chronic form, and no one discipline, including antibiotics, necessarily has the golden formula for curing it completely. The greatest successes come from an amalgam of combined therapies. With this book, I hope to offer insight into some options available. Please see www.OutoftheWoodsBook.com for recommendations of other books and resources, and take the time to do your own research as well.

Each of us is unique and each of us will have individual needs. What I like about natural medicine and the expanding category of integrative medicine is that they are tailored to that understanding—treating the person and not the disease. I share my success in these pages with you, to offer inspiration and hope. Please do not take this book to be a curative formula that will be duplicated specifically for you, but, rather, as a template to work from, giving you some options to explore in your Lyme recovery journey. I hope to open a window into healing options. Please tune in to the weekly talk show I host, "Lyme Light Radio with Katina" on TransformationTalkRadio.com, as we discuss all these matters and more with cutting-edge Lyme disease researchers, doctors, recoverees, advocates, and foundations.

Recovering fully from Lyme takes a great deal of time. Much more than most people initially want to accept. It also requires patience and fortitude. There are many periods when you feel that you cannot endure the battle, the fatigue, the pain, and the treatments any longer. It is then that you must dig even deeper, go longer, and hang on to your psyche more vehemently. This illness can be brutal. It will ask you to go places you never even knew existed. Faith, courage, and willpower are allies. I wish you strength and grace. You can succeed!

Acupuncture

Acupuncture is a three-thousand-year-old healing discipline heralding from China. Anecdotal evidence claims that this practice may actually date back five thousand years. Very little in this intricate yet straightforward approach to healing has altered throughout its history, primarily because the philosophy and practices of acupuncture have required scant improvement.

In 1949, Chairman Mao tried to eradicate the religious and superstitious mystical aspects of Chinese medicine and acupuncture, but when taken ill, his life was saved by this "folk medicine." So he allowed acupuncture to continue, but only as a less spiritual practice. In recent decades, acupuncture has moved beyond the walls of China into the Western world. Many people arrive at acupuncturists seeking pain alleviation, which is one of its fortes. The Chinese have relied on acupuncture and Chinese herbal formulas for treatment of organic disorders and conditions such as MS, asthma, colitis, infertility, stroke, insomnia, and more. The American Medical Association (AMA) has published a list of thousands of conditions that can be treated by acupuncture.

Looking at acupuncture in practice requires us to understand some of its philosophy. All living matter, whether a cat, a tree, or a human being, contains a life force or energy. This miraculous dimension, intrinsic to our existence, is rather difficult to evaluate through science. We all recognize that life energy, or qi (chi), as the Chinese call it, is vital to life, yet is of rather nebulous boundaries. Western science has been unable to determine accurately where life energy comes from and why it disappears at the time of death. But it certainly is real, even if unseen by the naked eye or sophisticated test equipment. Just as we know emotions are real, so is life energy. We certainly can't see the energy of anger or sadness, but when you walk into the room of one who is in the throes of such an emotion, you can feel it radiating from them. Qi is similar.

Methodologies from many Asian cultures, such as tai chi, macrobiotics, feng shui, shiatsu, qigong, and acupuncture focus on this qi force. Chinese medicine suggests that within the body there lie fourteen energy meridians that network the qi. These meridians run essentially in a longitudinal direction head to toe. Each meridian encompasses a pathway between various body parts, organs, and glands. Charts depict these meridians quite specifically. Practitioners also relate them to one of the five elements of nature as a way of describing one's system and the imbalances. You will hear an acupuncturist using terms such as Earth, Fire, Water, Wood, and Metal.

At various points in the body, meridian channels run close to the skin's surface, referred to as acupuncture points. When an organ is in a state of imbalance, these points exhibit a telltale signal via sensitivity and tonicity. These points have been empirically agreed on for thousands of years. Anatomical landmarks for where they are and unique functions that each point has attributed to it are undisputed in the profession. There has been some scientific research to determine noticeable differences at these points. Some studies have found a greater degree of salinity in the precise area of the points, while others have noticed increased electromagnetic readings. This research, however, is still under way and has yet to be completely verified.

The signs of disturbance along the energy meridians are rather subtle to the average person, yet practitioners identify them quickly. Chinese medicine relies on another facet of diagnosis: pulse points. Several pulse points are located on each wrist. These spots specifically correspond to the energy meridians. Through keen appraisal of the pulse points, a trained practitioner is able to access the status of the various meridians and the corresponding body parts. By correlating the findings, the practitioner is able to determine such bodily imbalances as anemia, heart disease, kidney weakness, and much more. Most of us marvel at the accuracy of these assessments when they are then verified by laboratory findings.

Acupuncture is actually a component of the comprehensive system of Chinese medicine, including herbal formulas and diet. Illness or states of discomfort are eliminated by unblocking, redirecting, and balancing the qi forces within.

Once the acupuncturist has identified your imbalances, fine hairlike needles are inserted into the corresponding acupuncture points. Unlike a hollow injection needle, these solid ones cause no pain other than sometimes a minute pricking sensation. They are inserted very delicately into the skin atop the muscles or joints. Joints are like rocks or boulders in the streams of energy flow. Various stresses, such as thermal, physical, emotional, nutritional, and mental, can also upset the qi of particular meridians. When such a situation lingers too long or is quite forceful, illness can set in. By activating the acupuncture points, the disturbed qi along the meridian is restored. When all meridians are experiencing adequate flow of the qi, the body functions in a perfect state of health and harmony.

Length and number of acupuncture treatments will vary, depending on several factors: acute or chronic condition, multiple meridian involvement, an individual's particular life force, and age. Chronic conditions typically require a series of treatments, while an acute illness may be corrected in one or two visits. Lyme disease in both acute and chronic forms responds well to acupuncture. It's both supportive and restorative, helping to build up one's energy, immunity, and wellness. Multiple treatments are necessary, though, as Lyme is an aggressive illness. Some people need months of devout treatment.

The Chinese medicine herbal formulas are numerous, some millennia old. These formulas will vary for each individual, depending on your manifestation of symptoms and the nature of the state of imbalance. Two people coming in with lower back pain may end up with different herbal formulas and have needles inserted in different locations, since one person may have blocked liver qi and the other may discover that his toxic colon is to blame. With Lyme, several formulas may be selected, as so many systems of the body are affected. Additionally, as the Lyme bacteria are killed off, the liver and kidneys respond well to strong support via acupuncture treatments and certain herbal formulas to help flush out these toxins. Acupuncture is a wonderful helpmate in this detoxification process, which is an essential component of Lyme recovery.

Some insurance carriers cover acupuncture treatment. This is an exciting step in the progress of our health-care system. There are a couple dozen accredited acupuncture and Oriental medicine graduate programs offered in the United States. Practitioners then sit for a national certification exam followed by state exams. The National Certification Commission for Acupuncture and Oriental Medicine (NCCAOM) and Clean Needle certificate course must be passed. State licensure varies from state to state. Some, like California, require separate exams for licensing. Each state also requires additional CEU (continuing education units) in order to maintain licensure. Your acupuncturist should be nationally certified by the NCCAOM and hold a current state license in the state in which you receive treatment. The NCCAOM can help individuals locate licensed acupuncturists in your area.

This fascinating branch of Eastern medicine can provide great benefits to many. Please do not gloss over its very capable workings during your journey toward wellness in tackling Lyme disease. I find it still to be a terrific asset even in the wellness capacity. Please see www.OutoftheWoodsBook.com for recommended resources.

Classical Homeopathy

Classical homeopathy is a comprehensive branch of alternative medicine that has been in existence since the late 1700s. The founder, German physician Samuel Hahnemann, brought to light two intrinsic principals, which are the cornerstones of this healing discipline. The first, known as the "Law of Similars," states that something that can cause a disease can also cure it. The second is the "magic of the minimum dose," which is the least amount of a substance to be used for curative purposes, but not to induce side effects.

Dr. Samuel Hahnemann was a research scientist working on understanding why quinine, or Peruvian bark, was effective in curing malaria. The suspicion was that its highly bitter quality was the essential reason. Hahnemann was not convinced of that explanation. During his studies he elected to self-experiment and began taking quinine himself. Curiously enough, a couple of weeks into this process Hahnemann developed the symptoms of malaria. This struck him as odd, as he wondered why a substance that was curing an illness could also cause it.

Hahnemann stopped taking the quinine, and the symptoms cleared up. He recommenced it and the malaria symptoms returned. This sparked the scientist's thinking. He turned to the converse thought process that if something can cause an illness to manifest, it could, in turn, be curative to that symptom state. Thus classical homeopathic theory was born.

Hahnemann devoted the rest of his long, illustrious life to exploring hundreds of common substances and their curative capabilities. He hired dozens of associate physicians and scientists to do provings on multitudes of substances, ranging from traditionally used herbals like chamomile and leopard's bane, to the more dangerous medical substances of arsenic and mercury. The cataloguing of these provings and studies done on hundreds of human beings is compiled in William Boericke's *Homeopathic Materia Medica*. It's a vast, brilliant piece of scientific work. Homeopaths still rely on this "bible" over two hundred years later.

Hahnemann was concerned about the dangerous side effects of taking too much of a substance, specifically arsenic and mercury, then used liberally for treating syphilis. This spurred him into experimenting with diluting amounts for curative work. Something sparked Dr. Hahnemann's thinking to shake or "success" each progressive dilution as it was made. He would start by making a mother tincture of a substance, akin to an herbal tea, then dilute it one part to ten and shake that mixture. He then took one drop of that newly shaken potency, which he labeled as 1x, and mixed that with another ten parts water in a new vial, shook that, and labeled it 2x. One drop of the 2x was taken and diluted with ten parts water, shaken, and became 3x. He continued this process of "potentization," discovering that the more diluted, yet energetically "shaken," potencies were faster acting and longer holding than the former one. So a 20x potency procured better results, eradicating symptoms more effectively than a 2x. This is the "minimum dose" principle of homeopathy. After the thirtieth dilution, no medicinal substance is found in the remedy, yet its effects are remarkably more effective than taking the original mother tincture—energy medicine at its finest.

Homeopathy spread like wildfire across Europe in the 1800s, becoming favored in the French and English courts. It made its way to America and across the Great Plains on wagon trains. Most households in the late 1800s relied on the homeopathic remedies Arnica, Lycopodium, and Rhus toxicodendron for an assortment of ills. The world's greatest homeopaths, James Tyler Kent and William Boericke, flourished along the East Coast at the turn of 1900. Dozens of homeopathic hospitals and colleges prospered in the era. In fact, the first medical society in the United States, known as the American Homeopathic Association (AHA), was founded in 1843, four years before the American Medical Association (AMA). The wealthy and famous, including the Rockefellers and Mark Twain, as well as the common man, found homeopathy to be gentle, effective, and reliable.

During the massive typhoid and influenza epidemics of the early 1900s, those who relied on homeopathic treatment fared dramatically better than those who turned to allopathic medicine. Homeopathic pharmacies abounded in all the major US cities well into the 1920s. Then, unexpectedly, things shifted with the advent of the Food and Drug Administration (FDA) and a quest to eradicate the "snake oil" sideshow charlatans peddling nebulous elixirs at fairs and on sidewalks.

Laws were created regarding patenting, a wise step, and a man named Abraham Flexner was installed to investigate the numerous "quack doctors" and lay-physicians trained at the knee of their father-physician or in the wards of a civil war hospital. Homeopathy, unfortunately, became decimated in Flexner's single-minded ambition to preserve only modern MDs. By the 1940s, homeopathy and natural medicine had essentially vanished from American life—pharmacies were boarded up and the schools' and homeopathic hospitals' licenses revoked. Only the Hahnemann Hospital in Philadelphia remained. Fortunately, FDA laws were passed regulating the manufacture of homeopathic remedies as standard over-the-counter aids, leaving them legally available. Still, with the advent of antibiotics and cortisone, both so-called miracle drugs, the pharmaceutical industry had planted itself front and center in our society, shoving aside all other modalities. However, doctors in Europe, Asia, and South America continued to integrate homeopathy with Western medicine, enabling a more complementary practice of medicine to thrive in those continents.

Homeopathy embraces many ideals. Respecting the wisdom of the healing force within is one of homeopathy's tenets. The body wants to heal, continuously attempting to right itself when off-center, using primary methods of discharge to purge toxins and emotional impediments. The essence of homeopathy is to honor these attempts by providing the person with a remedy that actually mimics the constellation of symptomology, not counteracting the process already under way. Suppressing or counteracting symptomology, as allopathic ("opposite suffering") medicine does (i.e., via decongestants or muscle relaxants), is oppositional to homeopathic doctrine. Instead, the simillimum remedy works by supporting and actually speeding up the healing process.

The two primary avenues of homeopathic application are acute and chronic care. Acute ills, such as sunburn, influenza, or beestings, are self-limiting conditions and readily addressed with a remedy, often in a self-help vein. Chronic ills, like colitis, fibromyalgia, or asthma, are treated by a certified practitioner at a constitutional level.

The concept of a "constitutional type" is another essential facet of classical homeopathy. Each of us is recognized as being born with a particular given constitutional blueprint or type. Classical homeopaths are trained to identify one's constitutional type by a set of qualities: body type, coloring, personality traits, and tendencies when ill. Genetic strengths and weaknesses in individual constitutional types are prone to manifestation of particular ills when run down or weakened. One's natural characteristics and specific symptoms are all valued as illustrative measures, guiding a practitioner to the wondrously compatible substance from nature that most closely energetically resonates with each person and his or her innate life force. A Cimicifuga (black snake root) constitution will readily develop depression, migraines, joint pains, and stiffness. Meanwhile, a Silicea (flint) constitution shows easy tendencies to developing colds, ear infections, chronic fatigue syndrome, cysts, and bowel irregularities, and often lack self-confidence and exhibit social anxieties.

It's critical for homeopaths to understand the person for who he or she is, as it's the person, not the disease, who is being treated. Discovering who each individual is and what makes her tick, how she reacts to the world around her, what inspires her, what deflates her, is the agenda of the homeopath. Constitutional prescribing helps restore harmony and balance within the individual, whereby the body is then able to right itself, throwing off the symptoms and illness of its own accord.

Classical homeopathy is still practiced essentially the same as it has been for well over two hundred years. Homeopaths pay close attention to the details of symptoms and their fluctuations. Observation is essential, as well as the patient's communication of his or her sensations and symptoms. The homeopath then matches the person and the remedy, thus coining the expression one knows so well with classical homeopathy that "like treats like." Allergy shots and vaccination principles have been borrowed from the homeopathy model of "like treats like." A minute amount of a particular ingredient is introduced to stimulate the body's own reactionary processes. However, homeopathic remedies are administered sublingually and are energy medicine, as opposed to shots and vaccines, which are biochemical preparations that are injected directly into the bloodstream.

Homeopathy requires two years of postgraduate training plus a pre-med background. Homeopaths are not considered primary health-care providers unless they hold a license in another profession, such as an MD, DO, DC, or LPN. Classical homeopaths can't give exams, prescribe pharmaceuticals, or make diagnoses. They will, however, make sure you receive the medical evaluation and care needed when indicated. Most have working relationships with allied health-care professionals, often in a shared office or clinic. The Council for Homeopathic Certification examines candidates for national certification annually. A good homeo-path must be an excellent listener, open-minded, and a keen observer. A strong memory helps, too, as homeopaths need to be intimately familiar with hundreds of remedies to pass the national exam.

It's a very tall order for a homeopath to pinpoint the one essential remedy out of over four thousand choices at the time of your first visit. Sometimes a few visits may be required before the perfect match is iden-tified, but then a whole new feeling of well-being is found. Symptom alleviation can be rapid with an acute condition, often even when the remedy pellets are still dissolving under the tongue, as with an allergy spell. With chronic illness, regained wellness comes during a span of weeks and months as the body recalibrates.

Classical homeopathy experienced a resurgence in the United States in the late 1970s, when Dr. Bill Gray introduced Dr. George Vithoulkas, master homeopath from Greece, to the pioneering collective of doc-tors, nurses, vets, and laypeople who had held the remnants of this healing art in a protective clutch. Soon other great masters from South America and Europe came to train these followers. By the late 1990s, homeopathic schools were reborn and pharmacies were on the rise. Today, commonly used potencies, such as 6c, 30c, and 200c (in which c dilutions indicate 1/100 parts), are available in most health food stores and even allopathic pharmacies, and large, high-tech machines make it possible to potentize remedies up to the fifty-thousandth dilution.

Homeopathy has not been studied at the scientific level during the technological mastery of the last several decades. It has ambled along, mostly disregarded as old-fashioned and a bit fantastical. Because it does not fit the scientific standards of pharmacology and deductive reasoning, much of our American medical system has tried to dismiss homeopathy as unproven and unscientific. It must be evaluated on a different spectrum, since its language and values are so divergent from allopathic medicine, being a system of empirical findings and data. Generations, however, testify to homeopathy's capable workings. Animals and infants respond to it unequivocally. Germany's, France's, and India's physicians are schooled in homeopathy.

Classical homeopathy offers highly valuable support in the treatment of Lyme disease. Individual remedies may be prescribed to treat the various acute symptoms that plague the individual, whether joint pain, stomach irregularities, headaches, depression, anxiety, or insomnia. All such states are greatly aided by the fine workings of homeopathic remedies. The ILADS 2013 conference even offered a lecture on the effectiveness of homeopathy in treating tick-borne illness.

The standard remedy for most all Lyme cases, to be taken at the earliest signs of symptoms—rash, headaches, body pains—is Ledum palustre, 1m strength, three pellets dissolved under the tongue, three times per day, for three days in a row. And get yourself to a health-care provider! Ledum can be used in older chronic cases, too.

The finest success comes when a homeopath can prescribe a constitutional remedy for you. The particular symptoms of Lyme disease you have manifested will help pinpoint the remedy needed. By supporting the system constitutionally, homeopathy help tends to heal Lyme more readily, and the other modalities—antibiotics, massage, and so on—hold better, too. The *Borrelia* organism can also be used with great results in the famous diluted potencies of "like treats like" capacity with Lyme. This is called a "nosode remedy," and needs a practitioner's expertise. It can be administered in vaccine-style use for those exposed to ticks frequently.

I, myself, have found homeopathy to be indispensable in the circuitous journey I have traveled in overcoming chronic Lyme disease. I truly believe that without the assistance of this wonderful healing discipline I would not have made the most obvious strides I have. Please do not overlook this effective modality. Internationally, it is a well-respected and utilized healing system.

Homeopathic remedies can be found in most health food stores or ordered online from the world-renowned pharmacy Boiron. There are dozens of singular homeopathic remedies pertinent to clearing acute Lyme (and co-infection) symptoms. Personally, Bryonia, Eupatorium perf, Pulsatilla, and Natrum mur saved my life! There are also wonderful "combination formulas" that contain four to eight low-dose remedies in synergy to use at a purely physiological, or what homeopaths call "clinical symptom," level to help with detoxification measures, fibromyalgia pains, neurotransmitter balancing, insomnia, and much more.

Nuances and subtleties make all the difference in finding remedies that are a "direct" match for your case. Seeing a professional classical homeopath (CCH) or naturopath (ND) who specializes in homeopathy is key! Many practitioners call themselves homeopaths. They are not properly certified. This is not a good situation. Homeopathy gets misused and misrepresented and is often ineffective in the hands of an only partially trained practitioner. You want a master, not a dabbler. This healing art requires vast training, a very astute mind, and someone with great perspective and finesse.

Practitioners can be found via the National Center for Homeopathy and the Council for Homeopathic Certification.

Symptom-Based Self-Help Remedies

As follows are a few "self-help" common homeopathic remedies to try for specific symptoms. The rule of thumb is to try a remedy two to three times per day for three to four days. If there is no change for the better, then this remedy is not energetically compatible with your constitution or symptoms. Just stop it and try another with a similar symptom picture. There are no side effects with remedies; they either match and work or do nothing at all. But, we do not take remedies indefinitely, only when symptoms are present.

All homeopathics are labeled by their Latin name, so they can be found worldwide at pharmacies, versus their common name (e.g., wind flower or pasque flower for Pulsatilla), which may vary by region. All remedies are to be taken with a "clean mouth," meaning no food, drink, toothpaste, gum, etc. fifteen minutes before or after a dose. Dissolve two pellets under the tongue, absorbed by the sublingual glands and bypassing the digestive tract. Some people note symptom alleviation in mere seconds under the tongue, others could require several doses for a change. Do not handle the pellets with your fingers, as they are sensitive to oils and fragrances and can become "negated." Just pop them in your mouth. Some people dissolve the pellets in two inches of pure water and sip the solution over an hour or so. Thousands of books are available on this wondrous healing art that India, Germany, France, and England have relied upon for centuries.

See HomeopathicEducationalServices.org for a vast array of self-help books, DVDs, textbooks, materia medicas, and more.

Ledum palustre: The "go-to" remedy for any tick bite, bull's-eye rash, and early flu-like feelings of achey pains. Another characteristic symptom is pain in the soles of the feet, especially the heels, often worse during the first steps after waking.

Take two to three doses of 200c or 1m potency within the first twenty-four hours of an embedded tick bite.

Chronic cases suggest lower potency doses of 12c or 30c strength twice per day for two to four weeks as a starting remedy. It is very well suited for *Bartonella* infections, too. Seek a professional homeopath.

Some remedies to use in a self-help vein for acute complaints of Lyme disease are below. Average use is a 12c or 30c potency, two pellets under the tongue, two to three times per day for three to four days in a row. If no relief is found then this remedy is not compatible with your system.

Bryonia alba: Right-sided body/joint pains, headaches, or migraines. Worse with movement. Wants to lie still. Often irritable. Fibromyalgia, arthritis, constipation, neck pain, liver issues present.

Rhus toxicodendron: Classic arthritic-type pains. Any joint can be involved. Worse in damp weather or aggravated by getting wet (even a bath). Pains are worse on first movement (mornings, rising from a chair) but ease off after being up and about for a while, often to digress in the evening. Restless feelings in bed at night. Neck, shoulder pains common. Skin rashes, shingle-type burning pains, too. Depression settles in over time commonly.

Eupatorium perf: A classic "flu" remedy where deep bone pains and upper back pain are persistent. Fevers or sweats can manifest. Deeply tired. Violent headaches. Epatorium perf is a strong liver cleanser and a favorite Lyme remedy of mine. Helps *Babesia* too.

Kalmia: Wandering muscle and joint pains (fibromyalgia, CFS, arthritis, or MS may be diagnosed incorrectly). A heavy fatigue and brain fog. It is a rare "pain-free" day with a Kalmia case.

Pulsatilla: Another migrating-body-pain remedy. Feel slight improvement getting outside, with fresh air or open windows. Company and consolation improve the weepy, sad, forlorn patient. Often a fearful, childlike helplessness is present. They crave warming comfort foods, dairy products. Many GI issues present: IBS, diarrhea, food allergies, bloating.

Gelsemium: Another remedy for a "flu-like" state with overall muscle versus bone pains. Back-of-the-neck-tension pains and occipital or frontal headache are common. Eyelids feel heavy. Drowsy, weak limbs. Occasional trembling. Irrational fear or anxiety, out of the blue. Clammy sweats. Diarrhea or IBS. Once fearless individual now feels weary and anxious. Common MS, fibromyalgia remedy.

Arsenicum album: A classic Lyme remedy. Lots of burning pains *anywhere*. Skin, GI tract, joints, nerves, muscles. Very weak, tired, yet restless. Cannot get away from the overwhelming pains. Insomnia. Pacing the floors or writhing in pain. Seizures, fits of rage, panic, fear. Oversensitive to "everything"—foods, medications, vitamins, weather, the wrong pillow, smells, etc. Nervous system feels fraught. Very useful for any form of neurological Lyme or co-infection. Even helpful to ease apprehension of traveling to or visiting a doctor. Usually slim, spare frame, or are losing weight when ill.

Kali phosphoricum: My favorite for CFS, collapse, bedridden cases. Completely drained, exhausted, hopeless states. Mental dullness/fog, depressed, forlorn, very weak, fragile. Insomnia. Strange nervous system sensations—buzzing, twitching, trembling. Tiring to "breathe." Homesick. Formerly responsible, usually hardworking types. Now cannot handle even a phone call, company, cooking.

Natrum muriaticum: Excellent for long-term, chronic cases that have been misdiagnosed, malingering. Patient is weary, filled with grief over so much loss in his or her life. Trying to be stoic, yet spells of anxiety, insomnia, moodiness arise. Low back and neck pains, migraines prominent. IBS, fibromyalgia, thyroid, MS, hormonal issues common. This remedy helps stabilize many chronic cases so that herbal support, hormonal therapy, nutritional therapy can work better. My observation is that a large majority of chronic (i.e., advanced Lyme over five years duration) sufferers benefit from several months on this remedy.

Another avenue with homeopathics is the brilliant work of the detoxification combination formulas. Helping the liver, kidneys, and spleen to cleanse is absolutely essential to clean up the body's terrain, allowing less burden on organs and glands, improving cognitive function, and allowing the immune system to run more effectively. See the detoxification chapter.

The product lines manufactured by BioResource Inc. and Mountain Health Products are excellent homeopathic detox support. Plus, they carry formulas for "states" such as inflammation, depression, or arthritis.

Extensive references, recommendations, and further information on homeopathy and Lyme treatment can be found online at: www.OutoftheWoodsBook.com

Naturopathic Medicine

Naturopathic medicine is a branch of holistic medicine that has been around in various forms over the centuries. Modern naturopathic medicine, or naturopathy, as it's more colloquially referred to in the United States, has been formalized through a standing medical association and practiced in our contemporary world since 1901. Prior to 1901, eclectic physicians, herbalists, and midwives practiced variant aspects of what we now call naturopathy.

Naturopathy has grown rapidly during the past thirty years. Sixteen states, plus Puerto Rico and the US Virgin Islands, currently license naturopaths as primary health-care providers, meaning these physicians can give examinations, make diagnoses, perform minor surgeries like lancing a boil, and address primary health-care issues. Numerous insurance carriers, depending on your locale, cover naturopathic medical procedures. Some hospitals grant naturopaths hospital privileges, enabling them to work with MDs in an integrated setting. Naturopathic physicians are considered to be some of the most solidly trained and diversified practitioners of holistic medicine in the United States.

Naturopaths go through four years of postgraduate schooling akin to allopathic medical schools. All the essential medical sciences are addressed, such as anatomy, physiology, pathology, microbiology, radiology, immunology, gynecology, diagnostics, and much more.

Throughout, there is training in therapeutic nutrition, Chinese medicine, homeopathy, physical therapies, and counseling. Although naturopaths rely on pharmaceuticals only when they are highly indicated, comparable attention is given to pharmacology during professional training so that practitioners' expertise is current regarding Western medicine's drugs and their side effects. Then the final two years include extensive rounds in an outpatient clinic setting.

In the formalized naturopathic colleges, many students choose to continue with a fifth year of studies, whereby a specialty focus is elected. This advanced training is available in obstetrics and natural childbirth, Chinese medicine and acupuncture, or classical homeopathy. The modalities of treatment a naturopath employs focus on diet and nutrition, botanical medicine, nutritional supplementation, bodywork, hydrotherapy, and perhaps other alternatives such as full-spectrum light therapy.

The philosophy of naturopathic medicine resonates with other holistic disciplines. Naturopaths treat the whole person, not necessarily just the illness, recognizing that the body's structure and chemistry are interconnected with the emotions and psyche. Emotional stress can have debilitating effects on the immune, neurological, and endocrine systems, triggering an array of unique responses. Instead of relying on drugs to affect the body chemistry and various ills, the restorative modalities employed include diet, botanicals, and lifestyle management.

The goal of naturopathic treatment is to find and treat the underlying cause of the patient's condition. Instead of palliating symptoms via the aid of pharmaceuticals, a naturopath attempts to regain internal balance and wellness, termed homeostasis, within the individual by utilizing therapies that do the least harm. Perhaps the most unfamiliar belief to some coming to naturopathy for the first time is the high regard naturopaths have for the body's innate healing wisdom. Fevers, muscle pains, or digestive problems are often signs that the body is attempting to reject toxins that have accumulated as the result of an unhealthy lifestyle or infection, or are consequential to destructive emotional interplay. Feeling ill can thus be a sign that your systems are attempting to heal you. Various naturopathic methodologies can help propel this process along, employing safe and noninvasive means to support the process instead of camouflaging or interrupting it. Neglecting symptomology, however, is not encouraged. If something hurts or disturbs you, it's important to tell your naturopath about this.

Prevention is also a key piece of naturopathic medicine. Much counseling is available regarding how to live a less toxic, more healthful lifestyle. It has long been recognized in various cultures of the world that our body is essentially a temple; that is why we need to know how to respect and care for it. Diet, exercise, and emotional fitness are all important. A premium is placed on avoiding potentially harmful substances such as alcohol, tobacco, caffeine, and highly processed foods, especially those with chemical additives, hydrogenated oils, or GMO food sources. Fresh, whole foods are supremely valued; organic, local sources are preferable; and commercially prepared items are to be avoided.

Lots of fresh air and sunshine, coupled with regular physical activity, keep our systems running smoothly. Our body is comprised of big, broad, capable muscles that need to be used often and rigorously. In today's convenience-oriented lifestyle, some of these commonsense basics are overlooked. Naturopathic medicine reminds us to care for ourselves when we are well and to turn to nature's bountiful resources when we are ill.

The Council for Naturopathic Medical Education (CNME) regulates the various teaching institutions in its capacity as an accrediting body. There are currently five fully accredited schools in the United States and two in Canada, graduates of which are able to qualify for the Naturopathic Physicians Licensing Exams (NPLEX). Upon passing these exams NDs are able to apply for a license in states that license NDs. These states do not recognize naturopaths receiving their training from the many correspondence schools that abound. The ND initials appear after one's name upon school graduation. If you are concerned about NPLEX status, do inquire of your practitioner.

Naturopathic medicine can be of tremendous support while undergoing Lyme treatment and recovery. In fact, my opinion is that a Lyme-literate naturopath is perhaps the most qualified practitioner to deal with Lyme disease. They have an ample toolbox of skills, and great access to finely tuned specialty tests that common physicians do not know of. Even if you are under an antibiotic-protocol regime, naturopathic medicine can provide many restorative supportive nutritional and herbal formulas, or bodywork modalities, such as lymphatic massage and hydrotherapy, as the body rebuilds depletions and cleanses itself from the Lyme bacteria and die-off. Detoxification is a critical step in Lyme disease recovery. The toxins that accumulate from the Lyme bacteria alone are enough to cause disturbing symptomology within one's system. The horrid brain fog and memory issues are typical of the neurotoxin brew.

As the Lyme bacteria are killed off, more uncomfortable feelings, energy loss, brain fog, and malaise can continue. Detoxification processes will help eliminate and reduce much of this symptomology and improve one's level of vitality and energy. Naturopathic medicine is a perfect avenue to resort to when undergoing detoxification processes. Detoxification can be difficult to try to manage on your own at home without proper guidance from a licensed practitioner. It's strongly encouraged to turn to naturopathic medicine for these purposes. Most medical doctors are not educated about the various support measures that can be employed for detoxification, such as herbs, colon treatments, skin scrubbing, sauna therapies, and sunlight therapy. Naturopaths are highly skilled in these modalities. Please read the detoxification chapter included. This is a naturopath's forte.

I was very fortunate to have a Lyme-literate MD who practiced integrative medicine and was knowledgeable as to using specific herbs, such as cat's claw, Artemisia, teasel root, and Andrographis to treat my Lyme disease. It's a rarity to have such a medical doctor available to you when seeking herbal assistance. This is where a naturopath can be of able service to those looking for herbal and nutritive support. A big part of the problem in many chronic Lyme cases is the very real concern of significant multiple-systems damage and depletion after battling the illness for so long, sometimes years or even decades.

The digestive tract can be a real mess, the lining irritated and permeable, the flora way off kilter, enzymes significantly depleted. This alone is worth seeking a naturopath's advice, as 80 percent of immune function resides in the gut. However, immune rebuilding, low white blood cell counts, yeast proliferation, nervous system exhaustion, hormonal collapse, and thyroid and adrenal compromise are all specific areas common to chronic Lyme that a naturopath will have valuable methods to correct. Plus many use state-of-the-art specialty labs that are better attuned to addressing metabolic disorders than the conventional larger hospitals and commercial labs, thereby helping pinpoint exact imbalances and enabling custom treatment unique to each individual, akin to the way Dr. Worthington did for me.

Please see www.OutoftheWoodsBook.com for current resources on naturopathy. Effective Lyme herbs, locating a practitioner, and supply companies are noted there.

Here is a sampling of some of the common Lyme disease herbal protocols thousands of victims find success with. We, blessedly, have some wondrous plants with Lyme-specific antibiotic properties, as well as an assortment of other herbs to tackle the co-infections of *Babesia*, *Bartonella*, Epstein-Barr, and more. Several decades into the Lyme crisis now, a handful of brilliant herbalists have established Lyme-specific herbal protocols for overcoming the infections, especially useful in chronic cases and dovetailing nicely with nutritional supportive aids and detoxification measures.

As you know, I never used antibiotics and I recovered 100 percent with the use of herbals, homeopathy, Rife, and natural measures. As one prominent Lyme antibiotic–skilled medical doctor said to me,

"Katina, I tell all my patients all the time, there is more than one way to get well from this disease," alluding to my success without antibiotic therapy.

These are herbs known to address Lyme and co-infections. But please, REMEMBER: Lyme disease is not a self-help illness. You need a skilled practitioner to manage your care as symptoms shift, inflammation rages, and the bugs play hide-and-seek. You need their lenses of perspective and nuances of which herb to use when.

Common herbs:

- Cat's claw (Samento is best brand)
- Teasel root (excellent for European strains)
- Artemisia
- Andrographis
- Lauric acid (retroviruses, yeast)

There are proven protocols that show significant success when adhered to with persistence (months and years), to choose from. Please explore these practitioners' work.

- The Cowden Protocol; found at nutramedix.com—Samento, banderol, etc.
- The Buhner Protocol; found at gaianstudies.org—Artimisen and more
- Byron White Formulas; found at byronwhiteformulas.com—A-bart, A-bab, A-Lyme, etc.
- The Zhang Herbs: these are Chinese herbal formulas
- PEKANA and Beyond Balance Formulas; found at BioResourceInc.com. These are homeopathic European superior-crafted formulas for detox, drainage, restoration, Lyme infection

I was on a modified version of the Cowden Protocol, meaning we administered the herbal formulas, but I never progressed to the maximum number of daily drops suggested. My system is so finely tuned that I made excellent progress at just half the amounts.

The product "Monolaurin" by Ecological Formulas (lauric acid) essentially "saved my life" by *finally* putting that relentless Epstein-Barr virus into dormancy.

Each of us is unique. Seeking a practitioner who is well versed in any of these noted protocols will be extremely therapeutic.

Rife Technology

Dr. Royal Raymond Rife, born in Nebraska in 1888, was a breakthrough microbiologist, with a state-of-the-art lab in Pasadena, California, housed in what we now know as Scripps Institute. He developed a highly capable microscope fifty times more powerful than its contemporary counterparts, enabling him to identify microorganisms that had never been seen before. Dr. Rife was able to prove scientifically that exposing specific microorganisms to certain electromagnetic frequencies resulted in killing them off.

Each organism, virulent or passive, has its own electromagnetic "footprint" of a particular vibrational frequency. Dr. Rife called this frequency the mortal oscillatory rate (MOR). He built a machine that duplicated and emitted the MOR frequencies into the body.

Rife had huge success in treating many cancers, typhus, and all sorts of other illnesses. His cancer work, in particular, was so highly praised that in 1931 a banquet of America's leading medical authorities united in honor of R. R. Rife at the Pasadena estate of then–Southern California AMA president Dr. Millbank Johnson to laud Rife's stunning scientific work and declare "The End to All Disease." Rife was a shining star, offering tremendous promise to society in the treatment of illness.

The tragedy that followed surrounding R. R. Rife, his scientific breakthroughs, the dubious sudden disappearance of his supporting colleagues, and the future of our understanding of cancer and its treatments is extremely disturbing and consummately unfortunate. *The Cancer Cure That Worked* by Barry Lynes goes into the details of the events that unfolded in the late 1930s through the 1960s.

As mentioned in the section on classical homeopathy, Abraham Flexner was hired by the AMA and was on the hunt to eliminate any forms of medical treatment not funded and supported by this organization, which was basically cornering a monopoly on the use of pharmaceuticals, a newly burgeoning industry at that time. Penicillin and the anti-inflammatory steroid, cortisone, had just been invented, true wonder drugs of the era, and were to pave the way for laboratory medicine to be the primary tool in a physician's bag of treatments. The Rife machine threatened this industry in an enormous way, as relying on electricity to treat conditions would not necessitate drugs and was much less costly. As we all realize, profits drive the progress of much of America, the medical industry included.

Two strange tales transpired around R. R. Rife during those times. One suggests that on the eve of a press conference in 1934 to announce the remarkably encouraging results of a 1933 cancer study with Rife technology, Dr. Millbank Johnson, the former president of the Southern California AMA, was found dead and all his research papers vanished. When an effort by Morris Fishbein to buy the rights to the Rife machine for the medical drug industry was unsuccessful, Dr. Rife's labs were burned to the ground. Awfully disturbing is the fact that Dr. Nemes, who had successfully duplicated R. R. Rife's work, was killed in a mysterious fire that burned all his research papers and findings. Another oddly suspicious fire completely destroyed Burnett Lab, which had also validated Rife's work.

The other version is that Dr. Millbank had a heart attack on the eve of the press conference, and his health deteriorated significantly. He apparently was the source of funding for R. R. Rife's research work, and these monies dried up, leaving Rife floundering and his colleagues in jeopardy to continue studies. Dr. Rife himself was harassed for years, driven out of the country, and, ultimately, apparently killed with a lethal dose of Valium in a hospital in 1970. His formerly supportive colleagues were terrified, and by 1939 all had denounced any prior association with him.

The good news amid the bad is that Dr. Gunner of Montreal, Canada, had replicated Rife's original technology, keeping something of this energy medicine alive. Many of our modern-day Rife machines, though still not FDA approved here in the United States, are a result of this fortunate measure by Dr. Gunner. The modern Rife machines employ electrode wands or plates, which are held one in each hand, or placed under the feet, to establish a circuit of the vibrational pattern that can be run through one's system.

Another interesting turn in the electromagnetic medicine story is that in the 1980s an engineer named Doug MacLean, who was afflicted with Lyme disease that did not respond well to antibiotic treatment, started experimenting with electromagnetic energy as a way to kill off the *Borrelia* bacteria. Unaware of R. R. Rife, he discovered the same methods for eradicating microorganisms. His more modern equipment, called the "coil machine," is considered by many Rife experts today to be the most powerful and effective on the market. One of the nice features is that the frequencies can be broadcast in a ten-foot range, so that the individual is not required to sit and hold the electrode wands for a lengthy duration of treatment, freeing the hands for other tasks. However, some more sensitive people find this machine to be too strong for them, and too bulky and large to handle.

There are specific codes in the Rife and coil machines directly aligned to *Borrelia* bacteria. Many other valuable frequency codes can be utilized, too, in one's healing efforts in recovering from Lyme disease. The inflammation channels, various joint and muscle pain channels, and the diarrhea, anxiety, depression, and memory loss channels are all available, as well as ones such as white blood cell enhancement, Epstein-Barr virus, mental clarity, and on and on. Thousands of frequencies are outlined in companion booklets to help individuals self-select appropriate ones for their body's needs (e.g., *Borrelia* code to set up an energetically inhospitable environment for them to survive in, or codes to stimulate gallstone decomposition, terminate a herpes infection, etc.).

It's quite an interesting piece of technology. Like antibiotic therapy, there can be a Herxheimer die-off reaction as bacteria are killed, making one feel worse before better. What is helpful, though, is that the detox, liver cleanse, and kidney cleanse channels can help minimize the effects of this reaction, supporting one's systems in this process. Drinking ample amounts of pure water is emphasized.

Outside the United States this technology is much more widely accepted and utilized as a valid method of healing. In fact, many conferences and symposia on Rife technology take place worldwide. It's a fascinating and amazingly effective tool in many circumstances.

Finding machines is not an easy process. The best ones are rather expensive—over $1,500—and there are so many various makes and models to be found on the Internet that it can be difficult to know which one to choose. To make matters more complicated, many companies are forced to close down quickly under threat of FDA invasion, but then open up again sometime later with a new name and model number in order to keep one step ahead. I realize that this makes the option sound rather cloak-and-dagger, but, in reality, the Rife technology is truly very valuable to many people and typically not harmful. Still, it is important to recognize that the Rife technology is not FDA approved and that all work with this equipment must be embarked upon in a self-help, experimental spirit.

Please see www.OutoftheWoodsBook.com for resources and links. Several in-depth books on the subject exist. LymeBook.com has a plethora of material available.

Note: The author does not endorse any machine or manufacturer. This book and Katina Makris make no medical claims about health benefits of Rife technology machines. The information is provided for the investigational purposes of the reader.

Detoxification

Our body is an intricate, fascinating complex of systems, functions, emotions, and brainpower, all working in synergy. A useful image is to think of our body as an individual ecosystem; the skin the outermost layer, with miraculous functions, systems, and musculoskeletal structure housed within. We have long heard, "The body is a temple." We need to care for our own personal ecosystem with fine attention.

I marvel at how fluidly our organs and glands help us adjust to weather changes, noxious fumes, a bleeding wound, or an invasive pathogen. We become stricken with bronchitis or food poisoning or the shock of a beloved's death, and our systems recalibrate and support us, always aiming to return to homeostasis or balance. Symptoms are the clues to where imbalances lie. We must honor these clues and share them with our practitioners.

When ill with Lyme disease and co-infections, an individual perpetually cascades through rotating sorts of symptoms. The inflammation cascade, hormonal imbalances, endotoxins produced, and assorted depletions set off so many discomforts. One of the four cornerstones to address for full illness recovery is the essential work of detoxification. Just as important as killing off the "bugs" is opening up our given systems of elimination, allowing for thorough drainage of the toxic stew

Lyme causes, as well as the "die-off" (or Herxheimer reaction people speak of) of particulates floating in the bloodstream and cellular tissues as bacteria, viruses, and parasites are killed.

Back to basics time now with this biology class refresher. We rely upon the liver, bowel, kidneys, skin, spleen, and lymphatic system, and the mucous membranes for cleansing pathways. Some of us in natural medicine refer to the skin as the "third kidney" as the sweat glands and pores eliminate fluids. Most integrative medicine doctors, naturopaths, and homeopaths often start a Lyme disease case (as we did with me) by focusing on supporting the liver, kidneys, and spleen immediately, and commence cleaning out debris, accumulated toxins, a sluggish liver and bowel, or retained fluids. By "opening" these pathways with the aid of homeopathic liver, kidney, and spleen formulas; herbs like milk thistle, red clover, cleavers, and marshmallow root; and/or supplements such as glutathione, activated charcoal, and alpha lipoic acid, many individuals note brain fog, acid reflux, fatigue, and assorted back pains reduce within a four- to six-week period. These gentle detoxification aids are reducing the burden your brilliant ecosystem has been laden with.

The research of Lyme specialist Dr. David Jernigan (Hansa Health Center) has highlighted that a key reason that individuals feel so ill, weak, nauseous, and brain-logged with Lyme disease is that the bacterium causes a massive amount of ammonia accumulation within. Our brain in particular goes into a sort of "numbness" or foggy-minded, apathetic state from the ammonia overload. Dr. Jernigan advises that the most effective means to reduce the ammonia buildup is with activated charcoal capsules (a favorite of my grandmother's generation), and the special properties of a plant indigenous to North America's heartland, the compass plant. See the website HansaCenter.com for more information on this plant and its uses.

As antibiotics, herbal antibiotics, and energy frequencies (such as the Rife machine) are introduced to kill off the *Borrelia*, molds, and co-infections, there are often very few or no side-effect symptoms if our detoxification channels are open and running efficiently. It is important to keep checking in with your practitioner and to maintain your detox regimens throughout treatments, to aid in curative work. Periodically, symptom clues can guide your practitioner to a spleen-, liver-, or kidney-support adjustment. The most sensitive people need fine-tuned adjustments.

Before I highlight some at-home, practical detox helpmates, let us note what a Herxheimer reaction is. Named for two syphilis experts, Dr. Jarisch and Dr. Herxheimer, it was noted that a worsening of symptoms, such as fever, chills, headache, tachycardia, hypotension, muscle pain, skin lesions, and anxiety, occurred after administration of antibiotics.

This Jarisch-Herxheimer reaction is a reaction to the endotoxins released by the death of harmful organisms in the body. Lyme disease, *Bartonella*, and syphilis can induce the "Herx," as the body is unable to release the heat-stable proteins from the spirochetes' death, creating much inflammation internally. Severe cases require IV fluids. Supporting our natural detox pathways can keep "Herxes" to a minimum.

What is nice to realize is that you do not have to live for the Herx reaction. Some Lyme afflicted believe the treatment is *only* working if they note a Herx response, but this is not true. A strong Herx response essentially means your detoxification pathways are sluggish or blocked. A wiser choice is to take a "time-out" from the "killing" protocol, reevaluate and support the detox pathways for a couple of weeks, feel clearer and stronger, then return to the attack tools. We want a good defense posture, meaning detox is working well, and not to rely totally on offense attack agents. Detoxification and attack protocols must work in harmony.

Another caveat of very significant note is the recent illumination on certain genome markers, or genetic mutations some of us possess, which perhaps set certain individuals up for very dire Lyme disease catastrophes or very prolonged journeys to wellness. The work of Dr. Ritchie Shoemaker, presented at the Boston 2012 ILADS conference by Dr. Wayne Anderson, is a brilliant educational piece on just exactly why some of us (myself included) succumb to Lyme disease so severely and others skate by with a mild fever, flu, bull's-eye rash, and a month of antibiotics with never a trace beyond. Visit ILADS.com to view this genius work and video.

Dr. Shoemaker highlights that some people house a genetic detoxi-fication flaw called MTHFR marker, which leads to elevated homocys-teine levels and inflammation problems, linked to heart disease, chronic pain, and detoxification burdens. If you have this genome, you will have a very difficult time detoxifying via your liver on your own. Your body needs firm support. Sometimes intravenous infusions are necessary. These are often the cases that struggle miserably for years or decades, until a savvy practitioner figures this out. The toxins are making you feel worse than the actual *Borrelia*!

Naturopaths and homeopaths are well skilled in employing detoxification measures. Integrative or functional medicine physicians have learned such tools, too. Make sure the practitioner you select embraces the philosophy of "detoxification, kill the bugs, rebuild depletions." This triad approach is very useful.

The common supplement agents for detoxification fall in two categories: the binders and pushers. Binders are activated charcoal, bentonite clay, milk thistle, chlorella, and green drinks. The pushers are alpha lipoic acid, apple pectin, glutathione, and homeopathic formulas.

Pushers help release toxins from cellular space, muscle fascia, connective tissue, and the nervous system, and help excrete them through the liver, gallbladder, and bowel route. We therefore want a good bowel transit time, and no constipation. If toxins such as yeast, bad bacteria, or estrogen dominance accumulate in the bowel, the lining gets irritated and more porous, allowing these offenders to permeate back into the bloodstream. This reverse process is termed "leaky gut syndrome" and many, many chronically ill Lyme-stricken individuals are caught in this muddy cross-current. Coffee enemas are an old ayurvedic practice to help promote good bowel transit time, pull toxins out, and clean up a leaky gut. Please seek practitioner guidance on this procedure and all liver/bowel cleansing "flushes."

The kidneys respond well to herbal teas and homeopathic formulas. Using a far-infrared sauna, BioMat, and Rife kidney-cleanse frequencies, and doing aerobic exercise that makes you sweat for only twenty minutes (don't go overboard and tax the adrenals) are excellent kidney/ skin aids. Lots of pure water is to be consumed daily. Flush!

Not to be overlooked is the lymphatic system, often *extremely* overburdened and inactive with couch-bound "Lymies." The lymph nodes make white blood cells deal with infectious microbes. The dead white blood cells accumulate and are filtered out by the spleen, a large organ under the lower left rib cage. The lymphatic system only moves the lymph fluids along with our body movement and circulation, or with the aid of reverse gravity. Staying upright or horizontal does not propel lymph. We then become plagued by lymph stasis, which leads to congested mucous membranes and makes you feel foggy-headed, bloated, and very fatigued or "heavy." Certain viruses, like Epstein-Barr, tax the spleen enormously. We want to get the lymphatic system moving and draining.

Viable methods include:

Skin Brushing: A Swedish technique using a natural boar bristle brush (obtained in health food stores or online). On dry skin, the dry brush is used in long strokes on lymph pathways, promoting sluggish fluids to move and stimulating the lymph nodes. You brush five to ten strokes on the inside of the arms (elbow to armpit), inner thighs to groin, and sides of the neck (ear to shoulder), all directed toward the heart region essentially.

Lymphatic Massage: Certain massage therapists are trained in specific lymph stasis techniques that help break up lymph accumulations.

Rebounding: Small mini-trampolines (approximately three feet in diameter) are excellent to promote lymph circulation. Please be gentle; the knees and back can be injured. No more than five to fifteen minutes of rebounding is necessary. Benefits are obtained even by keeping the balls of the feet on the trampoline and just softly bending the knees and sort of "pumping" versus jumping.

Inversion Tables: Actually going upside down is a means to move lymph. Children hanging from monkey bars or doing somersaults or headstands keep their lymphatics moving effortlessly and pass through infectious illness quickly. Static, vertical adults rarely go upside down except in yoga classes and such are rarely moving lymph. If you have been bed or sofa bound, trying to hang upside down or use an inversion apparatus will make you feel extremely nauseous, headachey, or sick. Below is a gentler, yet useful measure to employ instead.

Slantboarding: A sturdy, closed ironing board works perfectly. Place a brick or similar solid item under one end of the ironing board. Lay on the board, with your feet at the brick end, so that your head is lower than your feet. Remain three minutes in this "reversal" posture, then slowly get up. Some people feel nauseous or dizzy if their lymphatics are very congested. Repeat this posture daily until you can build up to ten minutes without side effects. Then move the ironing board on top of two bricks. Again, start with three minutes and work up to ten daily. Eventually you can escalate to propping the board on the bottom step of a staircase, then the second step, etc. You never have to get completely inverted with this technique. Working at a two-brick or such level of inversion is very effective, even over months of application. Some sit-up boards have adjustment notches in their setup. This can be another version of the ironing board setup.

Homeopathics: Mountain Health Products, BioResource's Pekana line, and Vinco Labs all make a spleen/lymph "drainage" liquid formula that helps promote good spleen function. Talk to your practitioner about these products. They were very helpful for me.

In summary, detoxification is a crucial piece of the Lyme disease and chronic illness recovery equation. Many cases plateau or never really totally cure due to the toxic overload a body is submerged by. Do not overlook this important piece. It truly is the turnaround quotient needed for many of the long-suffering, chronic cases, children and teens included.

Energy Restoration

Fatigue is a predominant issue in all phases of Lyme disease. Seemingly all Lyme patients experience some sort of fatigue, ranging from a mild malaise to an alarming state of collapse, wherein even lifting an arm or brushing your teeth feels impossible. There are numerous factors that contribute to fatigue. Most Lyme sufferers are looking for aid in resolving this unwell feeling.

Fatigue presents in the early phase of an acute case, when the immune system and its mighty lymphocytes, white blood cells, and phagocytes are being produced in record numbers in efforts to attack and remove the bloodstream's bacterial invader. Lyme is particularly taxing on one's system because the bacteria are initially introduced via what is essentially an injection (the tick bite), rather than via the mucous membrane entryway of viral colds and influenzas, measles, and pneumonia. The first line of defense methods of the immune system—tonsils, mucus production, vomiting—can abort such bacterial and viral invasions; however, in the instance of Lyme, the bloodstream transfer introduces the bacteria more deeply into the body, akin to HIV or hepatitis C. The immune system is immediately in secondary aggressive attack mode. This requires a great deal of energy—hence the significant fatigue.

Chronic, longer-term cases of Lyme disease deplete many valuable nutrients, hormones, and neurotransmitters. The aggressive work required of the thymus, spleen, adrenal glands, and more, in turn, induce secondary imbalances in the endocrine glands (thyroid, pancreas, hypothalamus, pituitary, and reproductive organs), since the entire endocrine system interconnects like an orchestra. Just as the woodwinds cue the strings in performing a symphony, the thyroid and other glands cue the adrenals or thymus. It is very common to find depleted adrenal glands, irregular peripheral thyroid function, and pituitary gland imbalances with chronic Lyme, all resulting in bone-deep fatigue and hypotension.

Because chronic Lyme disease and post–Lyme recovery and maintenance also require the rigorous work of so many systems of the body, the normal mitochondrial function in our cells can be compromised. Remember high school biology and the Krebs cycle? We learned how ATP (energy) is made by the conversion of fuel (glucose) into energy. In longer-term Lyme cases, this natural process may not be running properly, since the individual is not effectively utilizing nutrients. Some individuals have genetic malfunctions, triggering mitochondria dysfunction readily.

Supporting the immune system is essential in all phases of the illness. Early infections require vitamin C, good DHA oils (fish oil, borage, etc.), minerals (zinc, magnesium, manganese, and more), as well as immune-supportive herbs (echinacea, elderberry, cat's claw, and certain mushrooms). Naturopaths, nutritionists, and Chinese herbalists can be helpful practitioners regarding the first line of defense for immune support and which supplements to use and how much.

Chronic Lyme, in my opinion, necessitates persistent and experienced testing and treatment at the nutritional level. Addressing the often vast vitamin, mineral, essential fatty acid, and digestive enzyme and flora depletions is just as valuable as killing off the Lyme bacteria. Restoring hormonal imbalances and brain chemistry neurotransmitters is the domain again of certified clinical nutritionists, functional medicine, and naturopathic physicians. They also will be able to focus on inadequate mitochondrial function and glucose metabolic pathways, if appropriate. As with chronic fatigue syndrome, Epstein-Barr virus, or mononucleosis, working with digestive enzyme therapy can be very supportive. Dietary changes are crucial, too, necessitating whole foods, preferably organic, tailored to the person's depletions, and eliminating gluten and white sugar. Two great books, *Recipes for Repair*, by Gail and Laura Piazza, and Dr. Nicola McFadzean's *The Lyme Diet: Nutritional Strategies for Healing from Lyme Disease,* give step-by-step anti-inflammation diets and Lyme restorative menus.

Acupuncture and classical homeopathy both work with the body's internal balancing. Homeopathic remedies bring support to the immune system. When prescribed properly, improvement in energy is often the first sign that the "right" remedy has been found. Acupuncture addresses endocrine function readily, supporting the adrenals, thyroid, and more, helping to alleviate irregular sleep, immune depletion, and fatigue. The periferal autonomic nervous system has often been "damaged" with a Lyme infection, inducing low or fluctuating blood pressure, weakness, poor oxygenation to the brain, erratic sleep, and adrenal collapse. Termed the "triple warmer" meridian, along with liver stasis, a well-versed acupuncturist can help rebalance and restore qi in these meridians and optimize function.

Resetting the circadian sleep cycle, via pituitary gland and pineal gland support, can be a key step in working with the often abysmal insomnia symptom of Lyme. In fact, nourishing the brain and nervous system appears to be just as important as immune support in treating and recovering from chronic Lyme. As we all know, deep sleep is essential for healing, as is a comforting, gentle environment. Soft music and lighting, warm soups, nurturing, and peaceful time for inner and spiritual healing are precious balms to the ravaged nervous system. Pitch-black bedrooms and no electronics for several hours prior to bed are key to solid sleep. Love goes a long way in the healing process, too.

There are additional methods to help improve energy in the human body. The following suggestions are not scientifically proven, but anecdotal information and time-honored tradition have shown them to be effective through cultures and generations. It may by worth your while to experiment with some of these methods to see which can boost your energy. Books and CDs may be helpful in these matters, if a local class or practitioner cannot be found. Some of you may be too weak to attend a class. Mild efforts at home are encouraged: even fifteen minutes per day can start a positive trend.

Please see www.OutoftheWoodsBook.com for recommended resources and links.

Qigong: An esoteric Chinese healing system that promotes harnessing one's internal energy, or chi (qi), via methodologies involving static postures, breathing exercises, rhythmic martial art moves, and use of food and environment.

Tai Chi: An ancient Chinese exercise regimen of established, slow, continuous movements performed in a routine that circulates and raises energy (chi) within the body.

Reiki: Often thought of as similar to "laying on of hands," practitioners' skills are utilized to transfer energy into others, as well as to open or unleash areas of crimped energy within the client.

Yoga: Common now around the world, yoga's various postures (asanas) help promote immune function, increase energy, improve lymph and cardiovascular circulation, enhance optimal moods, and improve sleep. Philosophy and meditation may be incorporated in various purist forms of yoga practices. Most towns these days all house basic, simple yoga classes.

Rebounding: Very gentle jumping (only one to three inches) on a mini-trampoline improves the lymph and cardiovascular systems and strengthens the large leg and gluteal muscles, which prompts better mitochondrial and metabolic performance, in turn creating energy within.

Rife Machine: This technology offers energy-enhancing frequencies, including chronic fatigue syndrome frequencies, to improve energy. See pages xx–xx for more information, and review a Rife machine manual.

Bach Flower Remedies: A branch of homeopathic medicine, these diluted and potentized flowers were discovered by Dr. Edmund Bach to affect emotional states and have been in use since the 1930s. Their use in coping with Lyme disease (or other illnesses) can be profound. These remedies hold a fine attunement to energetic and emotional states. They are keenly sensitive and a great palliative tool emotionally. Many people note significant improvement for fatigue with olive. Clematis aids malaise and ennui in sickness. Gorse improves despair and depression.

Mustard boosts the already brave, stalwart personality who has stumbled and struggles valiantly against all odds to get well.

Finally, fresh air, sunshine, gentle walks in the outdoors, or placid swimming in open natural bodies of water (lakes, ponds, and the ocean) are all restorative and grounding for the over-sensitive nervous system. Nourishing the body and psyche at the emotional and spiritual levels seems to play a significant role in healing from the ravages of Lyme. Beauty, prayer, meditation, and the color pink/rose enhance endorphin levels, which in turn stimulate production of the "feel good" brain chemical serotonin. Good quantities of serotonin bring on a state of well-being, energy being part of that. Loving comfort and moments of beauty do great things for someone healing from Lyme. After all, healing begins on the inside, and creating inner states of harmony and bliss initiate a pattern of success.

Emotional Healing

T he physical symptoms and ravages of Lyme disease are tangible, though Lyme attacks different bodily systems in different individuals so symptoms are distinct to each person. Joint pains, headaches, fatigue, tremors, and night sweats are definable. Yet the emotional suffering related to this illness is often just as compromising.

People with a short-term acute Lyme disease infection, successfully treated with antibiotics, will not relate to the assorted and often overwhelming emotional experiences of entrenched cases. For those dealing with chronic Lyme disease, the illness can become the focal point of one's being, as it consumes the other aspects of living. Shock, anger, fear, sadness, betrayal, confusion, panic, frustration, despair, depression, self-pity, and dejection are all common emotions experienced by those suffering from chronic Lyme disease. Depending on the degree of impairment and loss one suffers, the array of emotions varies. It is normal to feel any or all of this.

Losing one's income and career can be a decimating event. Soaring medical bills associated with doctor-hopping, lab fees, hospital visits, medications, and supplements would overwhelm most anyone. Add to this declining health, lack of vitality, and an inability to function at a daily level, and fear and anxiety inevitably mount. Depression can set in when you become housebound and lose contact with your former social network and daily interactions. Partnerships and marriages can be very bruised and occasionally ruined when a life-altering illness moves in to your lives. The interplay and relationship dynamics change. Needs and expectations consequently shift. Some couples and families can make adjustments and work together with a serious illness, while others suffer gouging wounds.

The fact is that emotional suffering is just as real and pertinent as physical suffering. Therefore, tending to the emotional symptoms of Lyme disease is just as important as dealing with the physical. The emotions and the body are intertwined. Norman Vincent Peale promoted what he called "laughter therapy," and Mary Baker Eddy, the founder of Christian Science, taught "mind over matter," referring to the belief that a positive mind-set helps prompt physical healing.

Those of us who have walked "The Lyme Road," completely crumbled and trapped in darkness, understand the utmost necessity of tending to the emotional dimensions in order to reclaim wellness. Essentially, the Lyme disease experience is an archetypal Persephone journey into the "Underworld," or the shadow side or being, in Jungian language. All our frailties, past traumas, scars, and adaptive "props" come up for close scrutiny. This journey is not for the meek, but ultimately makes warriors out of many of us.

Those willing to embrace their willpower and an ability to self-examine, and let go of even their most cherished material and emotional possessions and patterns, will enter the domain, a vast openness essentially, of discovery, expansive growth, and the pure sanctuary of self-love. Belief ultimately is the most powerful self-sustaining emotional ally necessary to guide one to wellness—belief in your own ability to endure, belief that a higher power/God is overseeing your path, and belief that you will manifest the right people and circumstances to assist your process.

A quagmire I have sadly seen way too often is the tendency to fall "victim" to Lyme disease. Yes, this illness takes all your energy, brainpower, vitality, and lifestyle away from you. The physiological reactions it creates are not imagined. Studies have indicated that the fatigue, oxygen compromise, and weakness of Lyme is four times more severe than those afflicted with advanced congestive heart failure.

And remember: these are microbes that can be eliminated and/ or "walled off" in dormancy, plus we can mend depletions and damage. It is vital to *not* become the disease. You must reclaim your own vibration, not the self-defeating, suicidal, annihilating one of *Borrelia*. Wearing lime-green ribbons daily, hanging out all evening in negative, depressing Lyme chat rooms, will not help boost your emotional state, nor trend your neurotransmitters toward the positive. You must rise above the plummeting *Borrelia* drainpipe, the vacuum of despair, and *believe* 100 percent that you are not this disease, nor to be saddled with it eternally. Seek healing help!

Your physician may have some suggestions or recommendations for a counselor in your area. A pastor or priest may be of guidance. Lyme disease support groups are dotted about the country, and online Lyme blogging sites are accessible from anywhere with Internet access.

Additionally, some interesting and effective emotional processing therapies that have been developed in the realms of psychotherapy and energy medicine can be valuable tools for releasing the trauma, fear, and anxiety related to Lyme disease. These include the following, among others. Please see www.OutoftheWoodsBook.com for recommended resources and links.

EFT (Emotional Freedom Techniques): Developed by Gary Craig and now utilized in various forms by millions of individuals, practitioners, and clinics around the world, EFT is a simple, effective healing system that reduces stress, which is believed to be the precursor to much illness. Research has found this tapping technique to be effective for a broad array of psychological states, health conditions, and performance issues. Addressing PTSD and releasing negative emotions related to pain and illness are among EFT's fortes.

This modality can easily be employed at home by using the basic protocol to tap with your fingers on specific acupoint sites on the body.

EMDR (Eye Movement Desensitization and Reprocessing): A simple, effective technique employed by trained, licensed mental health practitioners to remove trauma, negative belief patterns, and PTSD from a client's psyche and body. Developed in 1990 by Dr. Francine Shapiro, this form of therapy is unlike the assorted talk therapies and closer in nature to EFT (although different in technique). EMDR recognizes that traumatic emotions, induced from an entire host of incidents, are stored in a part of the brain not accessed by cognition, analysis, or talking.

Using a bilateral right-to-left eye movement while thinking about a former event or certain feeling, the individual is able to reprocess the feelings in a new way and, in turn, release the old dysfunctional pattern, characterized by anxiety, phobias, OCD, insomnia, and illness.

Many Lyme disease patients are traumatized by the prolonged illness itself, as well as various medical happenings and their related physical, emotional, and relational losses. EMDR is an asset for helping with emotional healing.

To acknowledge the emotional component of Lyme disease does not mean that you are weak or odd. It means that you are paying attention to yourself and aware that you would like to make some strides in emotional as well as physical recovery. As trashed as you feel, please trust in your ability to heal. Take the step of courage and seek assistance. Read inspiring books, laugh with your kids, gaze at beautiful landscape photos, imagine yourself in one year's time, just as healthy as you aim to be!

Metaphysical Understanding of Lyme

Some people experiencing the effects of chronic Lyme disease may be interested in looking at the metaphysical aspects of this illness. Metaphysical healing unites the physical and emotional bodies in concert with the spirit. Each physical illness or condition has an emotional counterpart to it. Often, the emotional and spiritual components are overlooked, as medical interventions and daily life practicalities may feel all-consuming. For those individuals inclined to work with the metaphysical dimension, you may find this quote from my spiritual teacher, Dr. Meredith Young-Sowers, to be inspiring:

> *When the gut, the heart, and the spirit of the person are out of alignment, one is susceptible to chronic Lyme disease. Individuals struggling with chronic Lyme typically do not recognize their own true value in life. The remedy, beyond antibiotics, is a full body, mind, and spirit approach to restore one's basic relationship to the natural world, and to realign one's work in the world with one's true sense of love for self and others, all in alignment with Spirit.*

Take some time to think about this.

Advanced chronic Lyme disease is universally life altering. My own experience and research have shown me that progressed cases of chronic Lyme are situations that propel one into states of emotional and spiritual crisis. Change is asked of each stricken individual, whether he or she is hobbled at the milder end of the spectrum with persistent joint pain or fibromyalgia-type flares, or the much more dire circumstances of blindness, arrhythmia, or being bedridden in collapse.

The more debilitated and stricken people are, the more time has been created in their lives in order to reflect and realign with their life dreams and purpose. In some instances, one is taken completely down, stagnant for a long while, in order to get off the hamster wheel of his or her life, and start to look within. Learning to love and nourish oneself at the level of spirit is an intrinsic step toward healing. Often, individuals overcome by chronic Lyme may discover that the career or work they have done may no longer be the work of their heart. In these instances, a realignment with one's own deepest dreams and loves is crucially in order.

"The most advanced cases of chronic Lyme disease may arise in individuals who need to make the most radical shifts in their lives," says Dr. Young-Sowers. "It's not random that those who have the most to offer the world—those who are working hardest and have the most altruistic attitudes—can get hit hardest by this illness as they push themselves so hard, with little self-recognition." Is it any wonder, then, that multitasking women are most prone? Just as one would love a newborn child or baby animal, we must learn how to love our very selves with true compassion, through the tender and tragic mercies of this insidious and erratic illness.

Embracing our true love of self, others, and humankind can attune us to our true calling. From there a whole new life path is formed, giving little energetic reason for the illness to remain. Soon the treatments start to hold and the Lyme begins to recede. The illness has served a purpose by bringing us into true connection with self, the natural world, and its rhythms.

Yet the hardest hurdle may be yielding to this demand. I know it was for me. Stubbornly, I just wanted to hold on to and maintain the me I thought I was, the values I felt to be important, the marks of success I was raised to honor. Somehow, I felt it was frivolous to pay so much attention to my own self; after all there were others, more important than me, to save in this world. But, the Lyme told me something else: to stop, center myself, and listen within to just what it is I need and truly love. Like the delicate, gradual unfurling of a fiddlehead fern in spring, I, too, slowly unfurled into a new me, able to finally value my own inner gifts.

The inner gifts we each uniquely house are very precious. The ancient cultures and tribes of the world cull children at a young age, identifying their innate proclivities and strengths. They would train and apprentice them accordingly: weaver, healer, scribe, or warrior.

I was an artistic, creative, intuitive, nurturing child, rescuing hurt animals, sketching nonstop, writing poems and stories, acting out puppet shows, climbing high into the massive beech trees, my spirit soaring with adventure and my imaginary friend in tow. Yet, those painting lessons I begged for were never honored, and my intuitive inklings reprimanded as "prying" into others' privacy. My ambitious, Depression-vintage parents fostered medical or law school ambitions for me, dismissing my fine intuition and creativity as nonproductive follies. And, they were loving, generous, talented people. I adored them, but my heart's desires were glossed over. Post–WWII America was about achievement.

Only through the Lyme quest did I embrace the metaphysical process of this illness, the "time-out" it created in my hectic, high-achieving, predicated lifestyle, and how to reacquaint my own true inner self with my heart's deepest desires. The deep spiritual healing work I embraced, as *Out of the Woods* illustrates, revealed to me that my creative wellspring, enormous communication skills, deep connection to nature, and desire to nurture the wounded are my "callings." A doctor would not have been a bad choice for me, a classical homeopath was certainly better, and ultimately I found that becoming a spiritual healer and writer suits me best, for I am designed to cross the veil of seen reality and enter the sacred chambers of inner knowing and higher guidance with others. There we touch God's sanctuary and the keys to true healing. You, too, must honor the message Spirit is bringing to you through the Lyme disease journey, or any other serious life-altering disease or experience. This is not random.

My recommendation is that you find assistance at the level of the spirit. Often, very structured religions or, inversely, a lack of religion or spiritual access in recent generations has left many of us without skill or comfort in this domain. Perhaps a minister, priest, rabbi, yoga master, intuitive healer, or shaman may be available to you. This work I speak of involves different skills than psychological counseling. We are moving beyond the focus of intellectual and emotional analysis into the realms of the soul's purpose and earthplace in this lifetime.

We must explore realignment with our sense of the divine within our conscious selves. Ask yourself, what makes you feel safe? What enables you to trust your own authority? Where do you choose to put your efforts? Often these questions can be answered in relationship to how we love ourselves, others, and humanity, as well as how we feel empowered in life by our unique creative efforts and the work we bring to others. Ultimately, it is essential that we listen to the whisperings of our own hearts.

Finding our way through the briar patch of Lyme can bring us to a place of wholeness and fulfillment far exceeding our pre-illness life. After all, that is what the metaphysical nature of this illness is all about: transformative change. Just as a silken chrysalis harbors the hidden butterfly-to-be, chronic Lyme disease may be the container for your own rebirth, from which you will emerge with inexplicable new strengths and charms.

I applaud each and every one of you afflicted with Lyme disease for your tenacity, bravery, and inner beauty. Though you may be tucked deep within your cocoon now, in time, by following your heart's urgings and healing, there will come a day when you will break forth and fly on your own wondrous wings.

My Prayer

I ask for peace in my heart and in the world.
May love be my guiding force.
Bring no harm to me, my loved ones, or others.
Help me to serve for the highest good.
Let me be healthy and protected always.

Katina I. Makris

Appendix A:
Healing Intention Exercise

Lyme disease sufferers can feel bone-tired and forsaken. Many of us feel deflated, yet simultaneously overanalyze, wondering: What went wrong? Why am I so sick? Will I ever function at even half my former capacity? These mental records have deep, negative belief grooves cut into them. A new, more positive mental track is in order.

If ill health or uncomfortable symptoms trouble us, we can use the energy from our mind to support some inner changes. The conscious mind is the thinking mind, the part that makes decisions, collates details, and analyzes. This type of mental power is valued significantly in our Western culture. We school our children to use the left hemisphere of the brain, relying on logic, data, memorization, and science.

The intuitive or sensing mind involves the right hemisphere of the brain. Feelings, hunches, perceptions, and creativity are spawned here. We gloss over these skills too readily in our culture. Harnessing the energy of our intuitive right hemisphere and collating it with the logic of the left hemisphere is a valuable step in accessing the mind-body balancing conduit.

Letting go of runaway, analytical, or obsessive thought patterns and replacing them with loving kindness or positive imagery does not necessarily occur spontaneously. Like housebreaking a puppy or training a horse, repetition and encouragement bring results in the end. Be patient with your mind and your body.

The following self-help exercise awakens the mind-body connection pathway. It allows us to set the right-brain (subconcious) hemisphere in concert with the left-brain (concious) hemisphere, effecting a jump start to the physical plane. By prompting neurochemical changes with our thought patterns, we can, in turn, stimulate a chain of positive-effecting hormones, neurotransmitters, and immune responses.

Setting an Intention to Heal

Setting a healing intention is a time-honored practice to which most successful survivors are innately attuned. Some people naturally set intentions. Others may benefit from adopting such a practice. Anyone, of any age, is capable of setting an intention. All it involves is a clear wish, a statement acknowledging that wish, and, finally, a willingness to embody the intent at a visceral level. The prime ingredient is that this practice ignites the power of one's will. My training and personal experience as an intuitive healer validate the effective influence of setting an intention.

Willpower is an indomitable inner force. People who are able to connect with their personal will are able to achieve most anything. Working with willpower is an energetic tool beyond science, surgery, pharmacology, herbs, or other external adjuncts. This is something you can do from within. It involves connecting with your own inner resource of personal power.

Use the Intention Statement template below to work from. Fill in the blank spaces with words pertinent to your wish or goal. It can be modified in any way to suit your personal needs (any illness or state of discomfort can be addressed, not just Lyme disease). What is important in each sentence is not to omit the words in italic letters. These words and phrases connect to the will.

"I *WILL* be _____ (e.g., strong, healthy, energetic)."

"I *AM* _____ (e.g., healing, banishing, releasing) the (e.g., fatigue, painful neck, sadness) from my being/body."

"I *WILL* _____ (e.g., overcome Lyme disease, MS, heal com-pletely)."

It is perfectly acceptable to continue with additional *will* statements. However, whatever it is you wish to achieve, write it down clearly on a piece of paper and say it out loud to yourself at least once per day. Eventually, you will have it memorized. If you can close your eyes and visualize yourself as how you wish to look and feel, do that as well while you recite your intention statement. Imagine the expression on your face. Are you standing, sitting, or dancing? Where are you in your image of wellness? At home? On a mountain summit? In the stadium at a base-ball game? See it, feel it, and cement this vibration of the self you want to be in your conciousness. Perceive it. Believe it. Be it.

Listen within to the new mental music you are creating. It can be wondrous or perhaps unfamiliar at first. Once you grasp the melody, however, you won't forget the words.

Appendix B:
Additional Resources

There are many Lyme disease books, associations, support groups, blogs, and websites. Please see my website, www.KatinaMakris.com, for a more complete listing as well as supply resources for herbs, homeopathic remedies, and help locating practitioners in the various disciplines discussed.

Below are a few significant resources:

International Lyme and Associated Diseases Society; doctor training and info; www.ILADS.org

Tick Borne Disease Alliance; awareness and fundraising; TBDAlliance.org

The Lyme Times Newsletter; major support group network; www.lymedisease.org

The National Capitol Lyme and Tick-Borne Disease Association; www.natcaplyme.org

The Lyme Light Foundation; financial assistance; LymeLightFoundation.org

Lyme Disease Talk Radio; resources, practitioners, testimonials, inspiration; LymeLightRadio.com

LYME TESTING LABORATORIES:
IGeneX Labs, Palo Alto, CA; www.IGeneX.com
Clongen Laboratories, Germantown, MD; www.clongen.com

LYME LITERATE PHYSICIANS:
ILADS.org
LymeDiseaseAssociation.org

ACUPUNCTURE:

National Certification Commission for Acupuncture and Oriental Medicine; www.nccaom.org

CLASSICAL HOMEOPATHY:

National Center for Homeopathy, Arlington, VA; www.nationalcenterforhomeopathy.org

NATUROPATHIC MEDICINE:

www.Naturopathic.org

THE RIFE TECHNOLOGY

www.Lymebook.com
www.RifeConference.com

EMOTIONAL SUPPORT THERAPIES:

www.EFTuniverse.com
www.EMDR.com

HERBAL AND NUTRITIVE SUPPLEMENT SUPPLIERS:

BioResourceInc.com
MountainHealthProducts.com
NutraMedix.com
Boiron.com
StandardHomeopathics.com

BOOKS:

Cure Unknown, Pamela Weintraub
Why Can't I Get Better? Solving the Mystery of Lyme and Chronic Diseases, Richard Horowitz, MD
Healing Lyme Disease Naturally, Wolf D. Storl, ND
Healing Lyme, Stephen H. Buhner, ND
The Lyme Disease Solution, Dr. Kenneth Singleton
The Beginner's Guide to Lyme Disease, Nicola McFadzean, ND
Nature's Dirty Needle, Mara Williams, ANP
The Top 10 Lyme Disease Treatments, Bryan Rosner

Epilogue:
On the Lyme Road

O n bended knee I perch amid the hemlock boughs, stock-still, watching the pecking of a busy finch as it hunts for food. His tiny silvered beak dips and thrusts, stirring the colored leaves of the forest floor. Hopping, then darting, his eager work seems to be successful, as the bird flits to a branch, working his beak on his toes, then raising his face skyward as he swallows.

Soon there are two more finches, their summer golden feathers burnished to an autumn taupe, a hint of olive and subtle gold on their flanks. I hear their pretty voices, chirping as they dip and peck, clumps of green moss dimpling the dense woodland around us.

I have hiked and skied these trails over many seasons, cathedral-led in regal splendor, as heavy snows coat the conifers in Bavarian-style beauty, a muffled softness easing the swishing of our cross-country skis. Or, sauntering in with my children, as they climbed up the hillsides in a scramble of frolic, tossing twiglets in the bubbling brook. Now, the seasons meld before my eyes, my years in these northlands spiraling by. It is twenty-three years I have lived in these parts, a third of one's life in many instances.

A slight rustle ahead of me down the trail and I look to see Lucky nosing alongside a rotting tree stump. The finches take wing and I rise to join my Welsh corgi. I look down on my pant legs, instinctively searching for ticks. That fact is perhaps the most disturbing item of our lives—once a rarity in these most northern reaches of New England, ticks are everywhere now. We are all on red alert! Lyme disease has terrorized too many communities.

None of us can be blasé about the reality that we all run risks of being bitten by an infected tick. Even now, Lucky and I are potentially exposed. When returning home I will brush him thoroughly and do my own full clothing strip-down and body scan. I will never be casual again about my forays amid nature. In all honesty, I will be comforted by a twenty-four-inch snowstorm and subsequent suffocation and sub-zero freezing of the all-too-dangerous ticks.

Lucky and I climb to the top of the rise, up near the dinosaur-sized granite boulders, perched in a precarious tilt all these millennia, along a gentle ridgeline. We survey the crimson-clad forest, maples and poplars donned with jewels of early color. Eager squirrels scamper high in the trees, a musky leaf decay scents the air. It is pretty in a painterly way. I ease myself down onto an old rock, as Lucky wanders. Nature still soothes me, attuning my inner compass and senses, in spite of the dangerous ticks. My thoughts bend and cavort, as the wind does in the treetops. In these sensitive moments I assess that my life has become something I would never ever have imagined! It is miraculous what has occurred in these recent years, with lovely *Out of the Woods* by my side.

Who would have thought that the humble homeopath from the New Hampshire hills, once bedridden and broken, is now flying the globe, speaking to thousands about Lyme disease and the healing powers we bear? To fathom I host a weekly talk show, "Lyme Light Radio with Katina," on the famed *The Dr. Pat Show* syndicate—an opportunity that brings pioneering people, education, and dialogue to millions. That I have spoken at a rally in front of the White House, that *Out of the Woods* sits in waiting rooms in prominent Lyme physicians' offices, and that my health and vitality are like they were in my thirties are boons of unforeseen triumph! My world has expanded on so many levels, and I work hard, very hard, with intention.

What I have witnessed out "on the Lyme road" these last three years is too enormous to even begin to convey. I need another book to share it all. But, what I can say is that Lyme disease (tick-borne diseases) is ravaging the countryside, hearts, and purses of millions of people worldwide, and the suffering cracks open too many souls. This epidemic is surging and torqueing and I am passionate about helping change the future. How grateful I am to sustain my well-being and stamina amid a pace and responsibility level that is at times extremely demanding.

In my inner core, I know I am answering a "calling," and I cannot put my self in the way, but instead, I reach up and beyond, into the universe, and ask for guidance and protection. My life is no longer about me, but about something much bigger. Destiny has asked me to embrace my fullest potentials and I meet that challenge with gratitude and, even on some days, with pure amazement, for I am in awe of the synchronicities, the communion, the services so many devoted people are sharing with me and in our world.

Out of the Woods has taught me so much. This powerful yet tender book ushered me onto a pathway I did not predict. Little did I know I would be asked to walk into the open jaws of the decimating Lyme epidemic, and viscerally experience the crippling magnitude of what millions are plummeting through. The reality is that we are in the rip currents of a public health crisis.

Today, I walk with Lucky in the forests of our quaint New England hamlet. I am safe and vibrantly healthy. I juggle multiple jobs (speaker, author, radio host, healer), a teenager's schedule (yes, Eli is seventeen and driving), my home, and my own needs for reflection and creativity. Sadly, my partnership with Hunter ended. It shocks me still. That beautiful safe haven we created while nursing one another through terrifying seas could not hold fast when my "calling" to help the masses rang like a booming fire alarm in the stark night. I wish Hunter well as we move onto different paths. Our love was so enthralling. And, lovely Sarah soars onward, studying to be a nurse practitioner. Another healer weaving into our family tapestry!

My spirit is lit from within these days. *Out of the Woods* birthed not just a healing story of inspiration to others, but opened me up to something I can label only as magic. When uniting my practical world-savvy and guts with a channel to higher consciousness, I literally sense heaven and earth fuse as I walk into Lyme-stricken communities.

At times I feel like Florence Nightingale, holding a lamplight of faith and love, ministering alone to the deeply wounded in a dire time, with scant resources. Township to city I have traveled these three years. The groups who come out to meet me range from a small clutch in a health food store in Northern California, to over one hundred and buckling out the doors in libraries, granges, town halls, health clinics, and even an opera house. The pulse point I feel is that of alarm. The public is waking up to the reality that we have allowed a stealthy, unsuspect bacterial infection to pirate its way into our backyards and lives, and we have few known cures or even adequate diagnostics to face the grim fact that we are not safe. Lyme disease is a modern-day plague.

Globally, Lyme disease asks us to all hold hands, to reach into our pockets, into our hearts, and to the most brilliant minds, and coalesce our understanding and tools for mankind's greatest good. We all need to lend ourselves, even in the smallest of ways, to turn the tides. A single droplet of rain seems like nothing, yet millions of rain droplets create a flood. Our collective droplets of effort can induce that rainstorm we need.

How blessed I have been by the outpouring of cooperation and outreach across the USA. On a shoestring budget and grassroots efforts we have brought me to every corner of the country to speak. The Pacific Northwest to Southern California, from Florida to New England, I have slept on sofas and water beds, and been hosted in your homes and elegant cottages on vineyard estates. I am forever indebted and bonded to the remarkable individuals and Lyme support groups I have worked with, who so graciously help me bring information and inspiration to the Lyme weary.

I am humbled and eternally grateful when I recall the horrid years I was too weak to stand unassisted or even cut my food at a meal. Now, I dance and travel and distance-swim faithfully in the local pond in the summer. The Lyme experience is a piece of my history and my personal vibration has altered to an octave higher than *Borrelia burgdorferi*.

I call Lucky over and scratch his belly as he rolls on his back. He is ten years old now, but still an endearing, elfish fellow. I allow myself, in these moments, to perceive my work in the world. In my mind's eye I see an enormous arc streaming overhead as I swim into it. "Stunning" is what comes to mind. My life work is stunning!

The epic tragedy of what I witness daily with Lyme disease is wrenching. My heart aches for the single mother who cannot pay for her maimed son's medications, and the gray-pallored man in the front row, his arms trembling with palsy. The deaths, the bankruptcies, the medical neglect are grotesque. And, amid this soiled, ugly canvas, I still see beauty.

Your warm handshakes, your welcoming smiles, your lovely emails fill my heart. I have stood in your shoes and you can stand in mine. We are threaded through this illness and also with compassion. How many amazing individuals I have met on this journey: prominent physicians, ardent advocates, foundation leaders, cutting-edge researchers, media moguls, frail patients, and visionary thinkers. The Lyme disease community is filled with intelligent minds and very dear hearts. Each one of you is a precious jewel, and my treasure chest of life is beyond overflowing with riches.

This illness speaks of deep needs, and as a healer and messenger I am being asked to contribute all I can muster. Though daunting, I am also ignited with passion. Your fragility, your outpouring of kindness, your commitment to help others move me to keep taking risks.

As Lucky and I head back home, I muse on the vast tableau of places and the network of people I am now entwined with. Compared to those solo years on the sofa, my life is chock-full and ever evolving. The air is brisk. We walk quickly, striding with quest and purpose. Bits of blue pierce above the pine tops. The sun streaks in golden rays amid the boughs. My mind swarms. Every day I glean something new. I marvel at what opportunities I have been given. Inwardly I sing thanks to my spirit guides, for I am held. And, I am guided, a certain star calibrating my direction.

A particularly sterling moment crystallizes in my mind's eye: San Diego, the 2013 International Lyme and Associated Diseases Society annual conference. Four hundred twenty attendees from all over the globe gathered on lush Paradise Point Resort. It was a true honor to be conversing and dining with world-class researchers, doctors, practitioners, advocates, innovative thinkers, and many Lyme patients. My mind was abuzz with new information, exciting moments of synchronicity, and the backdrop of glimmering Mission Bay bathing us all in good fortune and promise for creating a healthier Lyme-free, or at least Lyme-controlled, tomorrow.

As we dined alfresco, Perseus Major, Venus, and the golden full moon bathing us in a fluid blend of companionship, and the poetry of inner attunement to mankind's plight, I felt at times as if I was living in a chrysalis of another reality. Like we were gestating and weaving together; harmonies, individual talents, trainings, understandings, and the Lyme experience, bringing to the table a certain gestalt, preparing for the birth of something very important. Palpably threaded in a cohesive tapestry, I felt a work in progress, there on Mission Bay—melding, blending, growing in proportion and form. The tipping point is close.

At ILADS 2013 I listened to interesting presentations on co-infections, glutathione pathways, retroviruses, biofilms, endocrine disorders, hyperbaric oxygen therapy, and much more. Practitioners left with many ideas and tools to implement with their cases, helping to rebuild depletions and attack infections, and to a veteran homeopath like me, the most *astounding* realization was that integrative medicine was being promoted as a key tool for recovery.

Thirty years ago as a newbie classical homeopath I was looked at as an oddball at a cocktail party, my job too weird-sounding for many to stomach. To find this cutting-edge, open-minded, medical-based health-care community gladly reaching to enzyme therapy, homeopathic formulas, detoxification methods, and herbs to kill bugs and rebuild damage was beyond my wildest imaginings from decades ago (antibiotics still in full force for acute infections and dire central nervous system issues). But, if it takes a public health crisis, called Lyme disease, to marry the two hands of health care, well then let it be! It was my great privilege to give the inspirational address at the San Diego Lyme Walk and Rally.

To quote Thomas Edison: "The doctor of the future will give no medication, but will interest his patients in the care of the human frame, diet, and in the cause and prevention of disease."

A particularly poignant moment occurred for me when a small group of four of us stood on the soft San Diego beach sand, city lights littering the bay and a giant full moon dangling overhead. Renowned physician Dr. Kenneth Liegner serenaded us with his marvelous trumpet playing, ending with a very moving rendition of "Taps," played in memorial for all those who have died due to Lyme disease. Our hearts loped heavily and I was deeply touched to be in such sterling company of dedicated people.

I left ILADS 2013 buoyed with hope. Brilliant, devoted people converged for four days, learning, sharing, and caring about this illness, the victims, and what they can bring home and utilize. Good folks doing good work in very hard times.

Meanwhile, I packed up and had a delicious waterside dinner with old friends. While walking along the bay, a wizened old Haitian witch doctor sat crossed-legged on the grass alongside the quay in the park, reading palms and telling futures. Ever curious, I sat down with the aged one with leathered dark skin, his glowing amber eyes peering deeply into my own. I asked for a "reading."

"I am in the presence of an angel," he spoke, and bowed to me, taking my hands, cupping them in his warmth. "You are a gifted and powerful healer, a soul older than my own. My skins prickles with your mighty powers bathing me now," his lyrical voice streamed.

I felt my spine tingle and was caught a bit off guard and was even a bit skeptical. The soft California night whispered in the palm trees. He sprinkled me with "Florida Water" and said, "You will not pay me for this time. It is not right. You are a mystic. It is my privilege to be with you now." I did not know what to think. Was this old man jesting, or on to something deeper than I even sensed?

"A man has left your side recently (my mate, Hunter, rashly walked out in June 2013). A family member, a man, died three years ago (my dad). But, do not worry, a very big heart will be with you soon. Someone grand and generous who understands you are a very rare person is coming in the near future. You will have five grandchildren. You are on a mission, like a saint or queen. Do not hesitate or feel sad for yourself ever. Your eyes tell me it all. You have seen the great mysteries of the universe. I can teach you even more, the old ways of African priests. You will heal thousands, even millions. Allow me to teach you. You are meant to reach many hearts."

I am sitting, listening, semi-uncertain, and beckon my best friend of forty-three years over to hear this. She sits near me. She listens, too. She smiles at the witch doctor/shaman when he repeats, "She is an angel, with a very big destiny." She nods a yes.

He proceeds. More prophecies are shared, some about my writing work and speaking to large masses of people. I do not know what to absorb. Eventually, with the cool night steeped in purple hues, I stand and bow to the old man. He hands me his bracelet, a worn woven wrap, and a CD of his own healing music.

"I pass this to you. Protection in the sea of life. I will pray for you every day. Come here again. I will teach you to *see* even deeper. Through thousands of years."

"I live three thousand five hundred miles away, it is impossible," comes my reply.

"Nothing is impossible. You are a master healer. I will teach you, even if I must come to where you are. I have been waiting for you to appear from my dream for a very long time. This is fate working. I must do a ceremonial cleansing botanica on you for more teaching to come. Come here tomorrow to take the rites?"

Is this guy a nut or truly a sage? Now, completely bewitched with eve falling, I shake hands with the crinkled one.

"No, I am sorry, I can't come. I fly out in the morning. But, thank you for seeing my true essence," come my words of gratitude. "You are a kind man, and very generous."

"I am only reminding you to *be* who you are," his Haitian accent, jumbled and colored with rhythms and melody conveys. "Very big work lies ahead for you. Do not be afraid. Your spirit knows what to do. Just listen to it. I will not push you. But, you will call me when you are ready to learn more. You know just what I mean—words are not necessary." He smiles, yellowed teeth flashing in a quick crescent. "God bless you, Angel of Mercy. You move with God's protection."

We walk away, or rather, I float away. I am anointed in ancient magic, while simultaneously steeped in four days of modern medical training. What do I think? How am I the conduit, the elixir, the carrier of Mother Earth's universal wisdom entwined with Western medicine's scientific workings? My senses swim. I am in semi-trance, all of this somehow stewed together within an eclipsing health crisis and a full golden moon riding in the eastern sky.

Nancy looks at me, grinning her mischievous smile.

"Leave it to you, to find a witch doctor in the wake of this weekend of left-brained didactics. Somehow, you manage to meld the two halves of healing, old and new, heaven and earth." We both chuckle, our eyes locked together in a smile, over four decades under our belt as soul-sisters. I feel spun upside down.

"I don't know what to really think of him," I say, wanting her opinion.

Pragmatic, poised, regal Nancy soothes, "He is correct. You are a powerful healer, he probably really does want to help you, and *yes*, you are positioned exactly in the midst of a health-care crisis with personal experience and professional knowledge and skills unique to all others. I believe his vision that you are destined for something important. It is just for us to wonder if you should take on his training? Sit on it for a few days, you will know."

I nod. I ponder. I sense. I want to try his ancient African healing magic. And, it all feels fantastical. Somehow, I try to let it all sift through me. I feel a bit off kilter. But, really, I intuit, I am just rebalancing. "Prince Alex" the soothsayer helped recalibrate me in that reading. After four days of science-mind and analytical reasoning, he brought me into my right-brain hemisphere of sensing, perceiving knowings.

Whether he is correct in his prophecies or not, it is okay. I will walk my path, lamplight of inspiration lit for those struggling on the Lyme road. As a messenger, I offer hope and faith and information. I "move with God's protection," though the footpath is never so clear.

Lucky and I round the bend to my drive. He dashes toward home. The large maple out front glows with yellow leaves, fine limbs reaching upward. We bustle indoors, ready for the "tick check" as my office assistant greets me with an endless list of daily email replies we must make. My life is in full tilt, and I reach forward with joy.

Step-by-step, day by day, I meet the sun, the sky, the ebony night, and the unknown challenges, plus the remarkable beauty of it all. We will amend the Lyme disease travesty. I am forever grateful for all whom I meet in this incredible journey of discovery and living. My gratitude is everlasting for an absolutely stunning second chance at life and groundbreaking work being shared. May the sun, the moon, and the stars all align for the highest good for us all, and may my heart touch yours with grace.

Blessings to all,
Katina I. Makris, CCH, CIH
Autumn 2014
New Hampshire, USA